Christine!

So much beauty bo... you.
It brings me joy to see.
Blessings sister.
I trust this will continue to inspire you in some way.
Get in touch when you're back in Leeds.

Love!
Robin xx (Hari Prem)

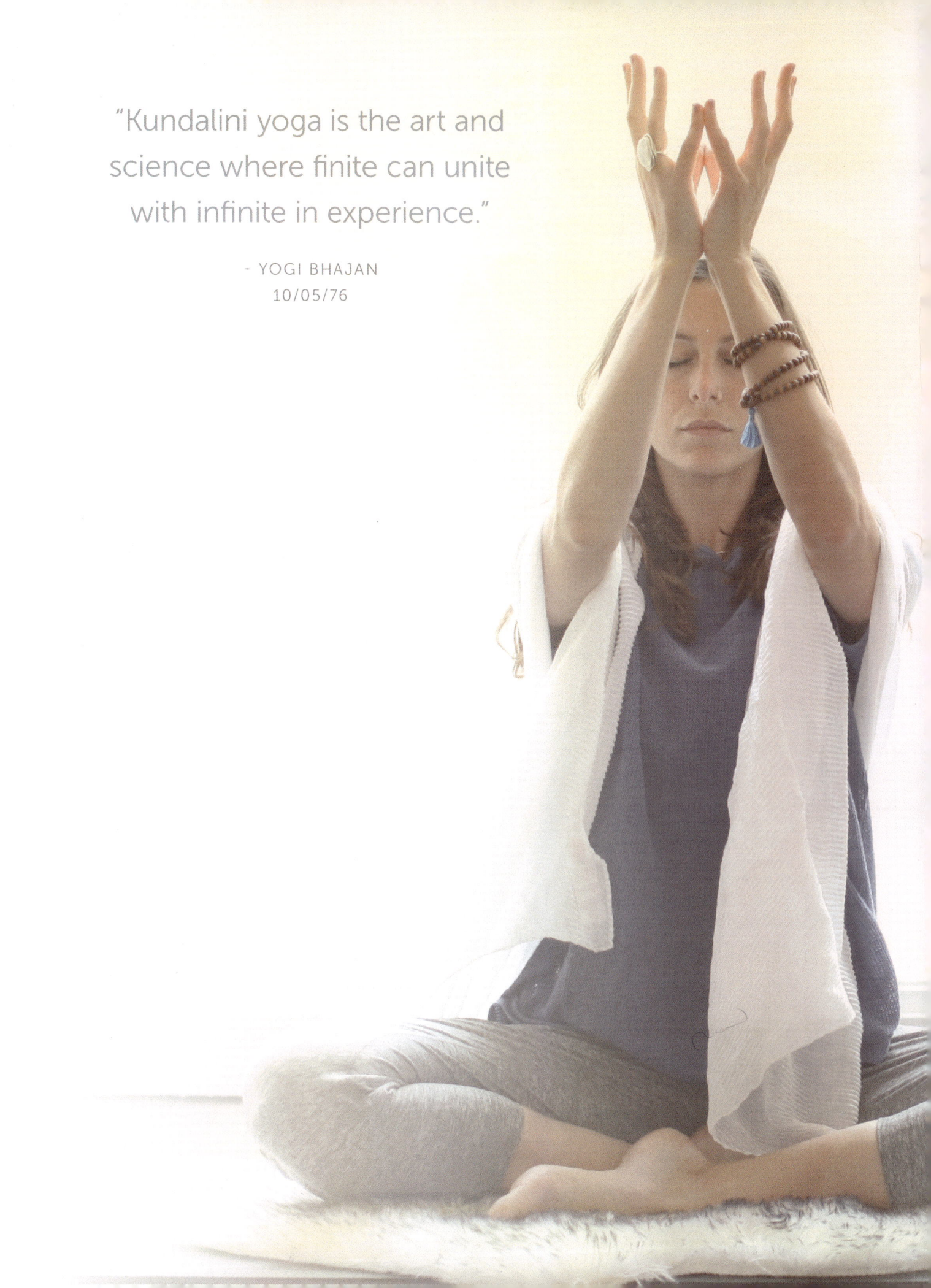

"Kundalini yoga is the art and science where finite can unite with infinite in experience."

– YOGI BHAJAN
10/05/76

Using a simple, Tantric Numerology calculation with your Date of Birth, you'll be given five key numbers – your challenges and strengths in this lifetime.

These numbers are your very own Tree of Life (roots, branches, seed, flower and fruit – your soul, karma, gift, destiny and path numbers).

These numbers also correspond with Kundalini Yoga's system of The Ten Bodies – giving you kriyas (yoga sets for change) and meditations to help you become more aware of and work through or with these challenges and strengths.

Cultivate your existence to the best of its ability.
Embody Your Soul Purpose.

#embodyyoursoulpurpose
@roisinallanakiernan

Disclaimer

The information offered (in relation to the yoga sets and meditations listed) has benefited numerous people but is not intended to diagnose, treat, cure, or replace proper medical care.

Before undertaking any of the yoga sets or meditations listed in this book, you are advised to seek the approval of a trained medical professional.

Anyone with pre-existing injuries to the spine or joints, those with high blood pressure, those who are overweight and pregnant ladies should definitely consult a trained medical professional before undertaking the exercises listed in this book.

The author (or anyone else involved in the production of this book) is not responsible for any adverse effects following the exercises listed in this book.

Credits & Copyright

Design and Layout
Joe Million (www.weareclay.co.uk)
Natalie Morton (www.letsdance.agency)

Photography
Ollie Jenkins (www.olliejenkins.co.uk)
Joe Million (www.weareclay.co.uk)

Copyright
© 2019 Roisin Allana Kiernan

All rights reserved.

All teachings, yoga sets, techniques, kriyas and meditations courtesy of Kundalini Research Institute (KRI). Reprinted with permission. To request permission, please write to KRI at PO Box 1819, Santa Cruz, NM 87567 or see www.kriteachings.org.

ISBN-13: 978-1548388706
ISBN-10: 154838870X

EXPRESSIONS OF DEEP GRATITUDE

First I thank my parents who I chose for this very journey. They taught me, through their own numbed pain, how not to live. It was following their deaths (only a few years apart) that I sought another way of being – a way of feeling; of vulnerability and of processing. Of course they offered positive attributes too – my Mother had a wicked sense of humour and my Father was creative and outgoing.

Secondly, I thank all Kundalini Yoga teachers I've had the opportunity to study with. To Nicola Heathcote who, with her trust and grace, gifted me with the opportunity to teach whilst still in training. Ishwara Kaur, for her disciplined and traditional approach, which I needed at the time. Karta Singh, for his more shamanic, physical break-through like servings. And Shiv Charan Singh for his subtle, intellectual and yet totally cosmic studies into numerology.

I also thank friends and family for offering their own teachings as well as every person who's shared the Kundalini practise with me, whether in class or online. We are all, always learning.

Great respect, of course, goes to Yogi Bhajan – the founder of Kundalini Yoga - a grounded human, truly being and sharing such transformative teachings. May he continue to inspire us through the ethers.

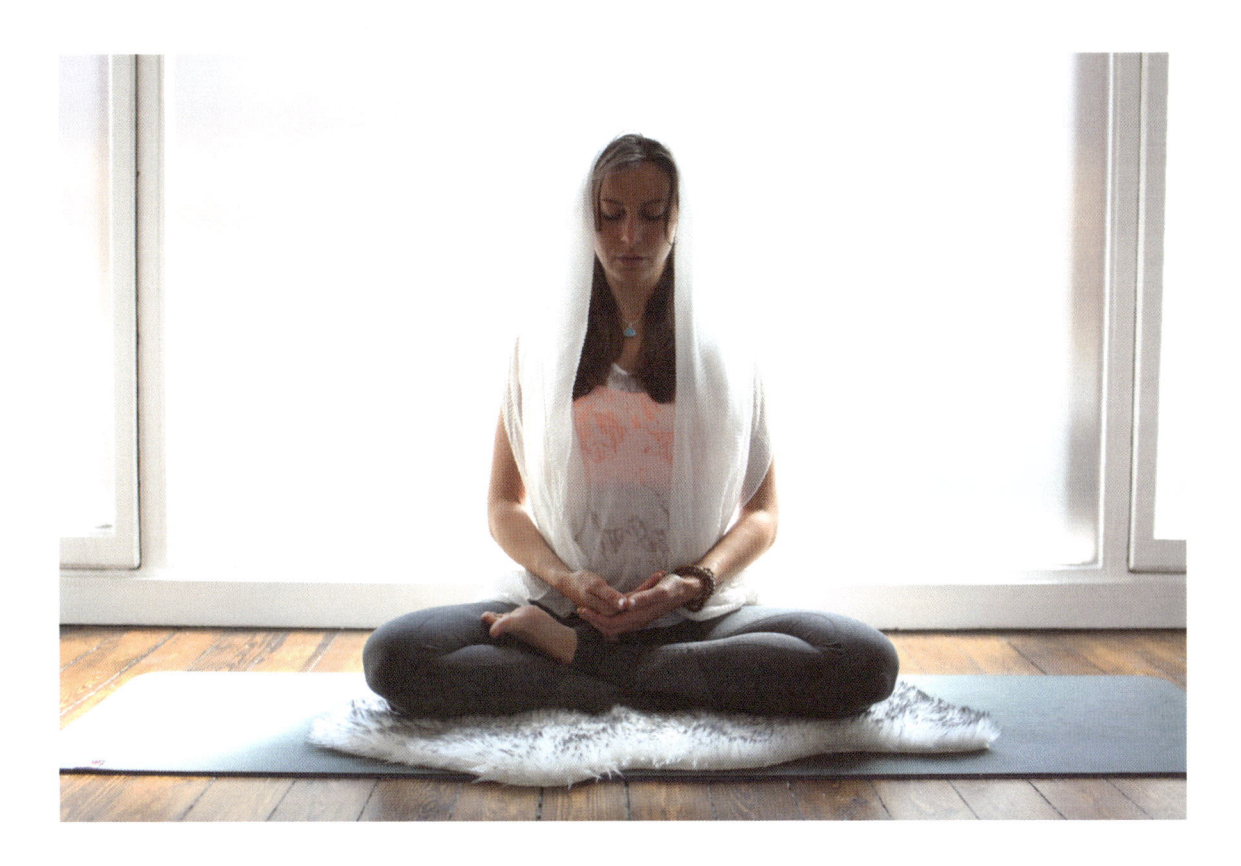

CONTENTS

Welcome And How To Use This Book 8
About Kundalini Yoga 10
An Introduction To The Ten Bodies 11
The Soul's Journey 12
Calculating Your Numbers 14
Your Tree of Life (Work Sheet) 15
A Quick Reference Guide 17
A Visual Representation Of The Ten Bodies 18
Tuning In And Closing The Space 20
Warm Up Exercises 22
The Sun Salutation 24

The Soul Body 26

Pranayama – Meditation For A Calm Heart 30
Kriya – For Balancing Head and Heart 32
Kriya – To Open The Lock Of The Heart 35
Meditation – Balancing Mind and Heart Unto Infinity (So Hung) 36

The Protective (Negative) Mind 38

Pranayama - Left Nostril Breathing 42
Kriya – For The Negative Mind 44
Meditation - For The Negative Mind 48

The Projective (Positive) Mind 50

Pranayama - Right Nostril Breathing 54
Kriya – For The Positive Mind 56
Meditation - For The Positive Mind (Sa,Ta,Na,Ma) 60

The Neutral Mind 62

Pranayama - Alternate Nostril Breathing 66
Kriya – For the Fourth Body (Neutral Mind) 68
Meditation - Shabd Kriya (Sa,Ta,Na,Ma – Wahe Guru) 72

The Physical Body 74

Pranayama - Breathing Into Your Ten Bodies 78
Kriya – Foundation For Infinity 80
Meditation - For The Tenth Gate: To Experience Your Boundlessness (Har, Har, Mukanday) 84

The Arcline 86

Pranayama - Meditation for Inspiring, Truthful, Deeply Penetrating Speech (Sa,Ta,Na,Ma) 90
Kriya – Adjust Your Flow With The Four U's 92
Meditation For The Arcline And To Clear The Karmas (Wahe Guru, Wahe Jio) 94

The Aura 96

Pranayama - Aura Builder 100
Kriya – For S.A.D And Depression 102
Meditation - The Divine Shield For Protection And Positivity (Maaa) 108

The Pranic Body 110

Pranayama - Breath Of Fire Expansion 114
Kriya – Preparatory Exercises For Lungs, Magnetic Field And Deep Meditation 116
Meditation - Deep Meditation 122

The Subtle Body 124

Pranayama - Meditation On The White Swan 128
Kriya – To Clarify The Subtle Body (Har) 130
Kriya – Laya Yoga For Intuition And The Power To Heal (Ek Ong Kar) 131
Meditation - Antar Naad Mudra (Sa,Re,Sa,Sa) 134

The Radiant Body 136

Pranayama - Archer Pose (Warrior 2) 140
Kriya – For The Radiant Body 142
Meditation - To Develop The Radiant Body (Ajai Alai) 146

The All-In-One (Relationship) Body 148

Pranayama - Seven-Wave Sat Nam 152
Kriya – Awakening To Your Ten Bodies 154
Meditation - Laya Yoga (Ek Ong Kar) 160

About The Author 162
Quick Reference Guide 163
Resources 164
Glossary 166

WELCOME

My aim with this book is to offer an accessible understanding and embodied exploration of your Soul's Purpose.

Using a simple, Tantric Numerology calculation with your Date of Birth, you'll be given five key numbers – your strengths and challenges in this lifetime. These numbers are your very own Tree of Life (roots, branches, seed, flower, and fruit – your soul, karma, gift, destiny, and path numbers). Numbers which correspond with Kundalini Yoga's system of The Ten Bodies – giving you kriyas (yoga sets for change) and meditations to help you become more aware of and work through these strengths and challenges.

Your Soul Purpose/Tree of Life numbers are a lifelong lesson, as written in the palm of your hand when your soul chose to incarnate in your body. I am so excited for you and know that your path will find its own way but I've also listed some suggestions to support your use of this book as a guide.

Kundalini Yoga is designed to support your soul connection. It's a powerfully transformative and supportive practice, but when I first started teaching the numerous Kriyas (sets for change) felt overwhelming. I knew back then that offering workbooks like this would be a handy gift for people - to explore the teachings themselves and to share in classes. So, over the years, I've tested this and other courses in my own classes and am now offering them to you.

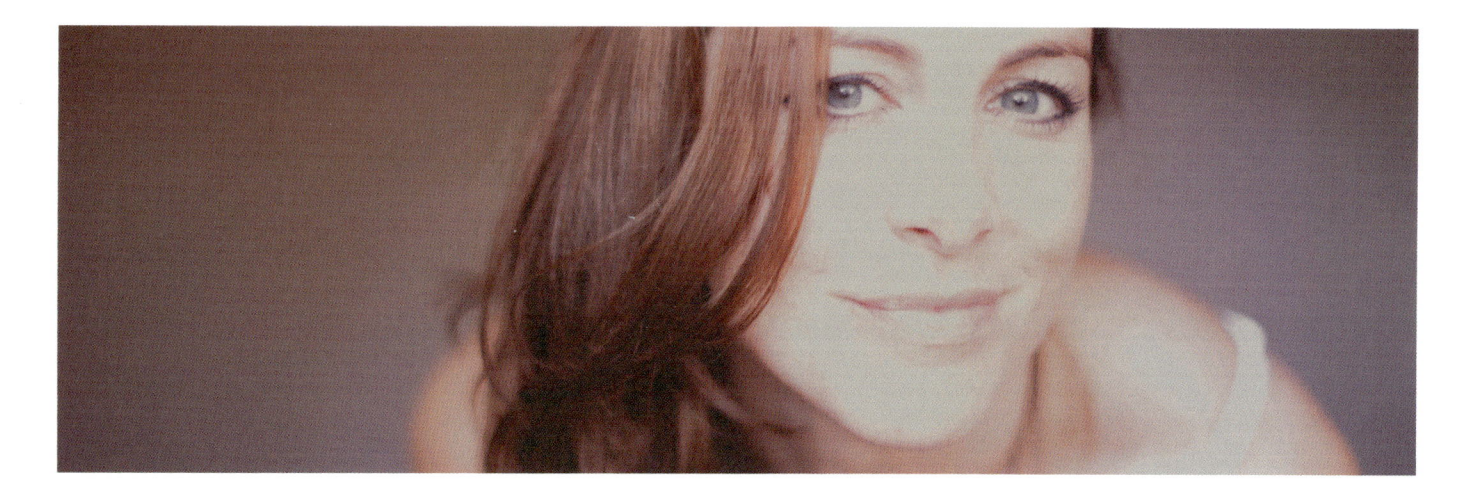

HOW TO USE THIS BOOK

I have taken great care with the lay out of this book, which is designed to guide you gently in an understanding of your Soul's Tree of Life numbers in association with The Ten Bodies system of Kundalini Yoga. As such, I would suggest that you follow the introductory pages in the order they are listed. There's a Resources page at the back of the book too. That details my own research into Yogi Bhajan's teachings of The Ten Bodies and Shiv Charan Singh's associated offerings on Numerology or Karam Kriya, as he calls it.

The first information you'll find in this book is an introduction to The Ten Bodies, followed by an explanation of The Soul's Journey of awakening through the bodies or numbers, a calculation sheet to work out your own Tree of Life numbers, and a Quick Reference guide to each body. I've also then created what I believe offers a visual representation of The Ten Bodies – my way of helping you understand and start to experience the intangible.

Each of The Ten Bodies have their own chapter, complete with an Introduction, Pranayama (breathing exercise), Kriya (set for change) and Meditation. They are laid out in this way, so that you have a full class for each body. Each aspect (the Pranayama, Kriya or Meditation) can also be explored individually.

Kundalini Yoga classes begin by 'tuning in' with the Adi Mantra; connecting to your higher, Infinite, Soul self, and all those connected to the practise (explained in more detail on page 20). I encourage you to explore and utilise this 'tuning in' meditation, because it sets the intention for the whole practise – that this is for you to connect deeper with you. After tuning in, Kundalini Yoga classes will often include a warm up (also offered in this book), Pranayama, Kriya, relaxation time and then a Meditation, before tuning out with Sat Nam (again explained on page 20).

In terms of your experiential use with The Ten Bodies information and exercises, just explore. Do your calculations, work out your Tree of Life, read, try an exercise and feel the responses, both to the physical and intellectual. You might like to go through each body methodically, or jump straight into those associated with your numbers – all is fine. Often it's the aspects you find most challenging that will offer the greatest breakthroughs but take your time with it.

All these bodies work together as a whole – they are inter-connected. Just because some bodies may be your challenges or strengths, doesn't mean the others are less important. I suggest working your way through them all – maybe starting with your challenges. You might immediately recognise your strengths anyway, so you could leave them until last, perhaps drawing on them specifically in times of need.

That said, a daily practise is when the real transformation occurs – 40 consecutive days of thev same kriya or meditation will break a habit, 90 will form a new one and 1000 will master something; miss a day and you start again. You can feel the benefits after only one session but commitment is needed to make lasting changes. I have worked closely with friends, set up social media groups and run courses to support this daily transformational process. You too can do the same.

Be compassionate with yourself though – we are all imperfectly perfect, no matter what stage we are at in our own personal journey. Have gratitude, simply for your body and breath – for life.

Teachers – I offer this book as a guide for you to share from. You could work through each body as a course or offer workshops on The Soul Body, The Mind, The Physical Body or the Energy Bodies, for example. I recommend exploring each set and meditation for yourself first, so that you can bring your own experience into the lessons too.

I've endeavoured to explain most terms as they arise through the book. More detailed explanations are listed in the Glossary at the back of the book.

As ever, I'm here to support your journey, so please get in touch if you have any further questions. I'm always keen to hear how you're getting on with the teachings too. Many of my students have gone on to become teachers themselves and this might be something you could explore in the future.

All love,

Róisín xx

ABOUT KUNDALINI YOGA

Kundalini Yoga, as taught by Yogi Bhajan® (shown below), was brought to California by the main man himself in the '60s. He saw the hippies dropping out of a society they didn't want and felt helpless to change – so he offered them this practise of transformation. In that sense, Kundalini Yoga is relatively new to the West, but it's growing and is designed for these changing times.

Yogi Bhajan's aim was to support people in the shift from our Piscean to Aquarian Age – from a time of hierarchy into equality. An astrological shift that happens every 2000 years and has been foreseen by many ancient people, including the Hindus, Egyptians, Maya and Hopis. Most of you will have heard of something going on around December 21, 2012 (please see resources for further information on this date) – when we entered this new age. We're in a transformational, tumultuous time, with a pressure that's necessary for change. But positive change is coming and Kundalini Yoga is specifically designed to support you through the process.

Also known as The Yoga of Awareness, for its ability to bring insight into the practitioner on a deep psychological level, Kundalini Yoga is potent and powerful and will shake you up – in a good way. It gets you physically and mentally fit and fast.

Every kriya (or set for change) and meditation is designed to produce a specific response within the body. The exercises in a Kundalini Yoga set or meditation may involve repetitive or holding postures, some are dynamic, others very still, some use mantra, others visualisations. Every kriya or meditation is different in this way.

'Kundalini' literally means 'the lock of hair of the beloved'. It is a massive dormant energy that holds your full potential. Kundalini Yoga works to uncoil that potential – to awaken and rise it up from the base of your spine. To help you Embody Your Soul Purpose.

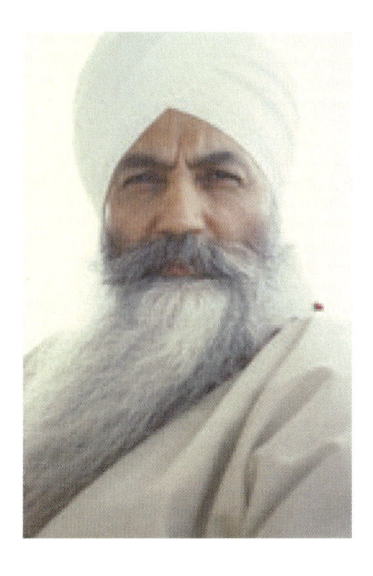

INTRODUCTION TO THE TEN BODIES

You are not one simple functioning instrument, rather a symphony that could – if you let it – be plucked and keyed into harmony by ten bodies - one physical, three mental and six energetic. Through them you can harness your strengths, overcome your challenges, learn to adapt your reactionary tendencies and start to trust your intuition.

Just as a symphony of instruments work together to create harmony, so too do your ten bodies. When one is out of balance then the rest are affected. Life, or energy, needs to flow, so a block in one of these bodies will eventually lead to stagnation and, ultimately, illness. Maintaining balance in the body leads to a healthy and happy life.

The Ten Bodies offer a way of understanding and cleansing yourself – physically and energetically - so you can be healthy and happy.

A simple calculation (shown on page 14), using your Date of Birth with Tantric Numerology, gives you five key numbers, or bodies, showing your strengths and challenges in this lifetime – your very own Tree of Life (each key number relates to an aspect of your tree).

NUMEROLOGY UNITES ALL

Of course, there are varying methods of interpretation – the Egyptians, Chinese and Jewish people all have their ways – but they all interlink too. In fact, numbers are the backbone of all.

There is so much further you can go with these studies and real understanding takes time. Mentally you might be dubious but some of 'your numbers' will ring true. When you start working with them then you'll see. Try it on friends and family too – you may be able to see them in the numbers better than they can themselves.

The Ten Sikh Gurus are directly related to The Ten Bodies system (Yogi Bhajan was a Sikh) – their lives represent archetypes for each of the bodies. Also, Shiv Charan Singh has a school and several books specifically dedicated to what he calls the spiritual science of numerology or Karam Kriya. Kundalini Yoga itself can be taken in many further directions too. Welcome to a whole new world of awareness!

THE SOUL'S JOURNEY

The Ten Bodies all work together – they are all parts of you – but each also marks the consecutive progression of your soul's journey. Over the next couple of pages you'll be able to work out your Tree of Life numbers and read through a quick overview of each body. But first, here's a quick break down of the soul's journey of awakening, as shown through the progression of the bodies and their numbers.

1. The Soul Body

The Soul Body contains the essence of a person made manifest in the body. It is the very first step in this lifetime. But are you No.1 or one of all?

2. The Protective (Negative) Mind

In two we find duality; the realisation that although each person contains a soul, each person is also an individual. In this respect the second body – The Protective (Negative) Mind – creates separation, which paradoxically is all about relationship. It instils a longing to return to the soul's infinite connection; a need.

3. The Projective (Positive) Mind

In three we're given an opportunity for structure again - a complete cycle or shape; a triangle - removing separation and bringing equality. The Projective (Positive) Mind brings optimism to our lives and the understanding that we are all individually responsible for re-connecting. Balance, or equality, rather than control is key though.

4. The Neutral (Meditative) Mind

A square has four equal sides, which is symbolic of this body, for it is at this stage that the soul begins to awaken to the Infinite once more. An awakening that brings the acceptance that each individual is infinitely connected, whilst also paradoxically being an individual. Will you allow yourself to breathe fully in and out of this realisation, drop your protection and/or control and find the balance of The Neutral Mind?

5. The Physical Body

Five is the balance point – the half way mark. Having understood the connection, the soul must then find the way to communicate this truth; to itself and others. The fifth, Physical Body, can be our greatest guide, if only we listen (to ourselves and others), with all five senses.

6. The Arcline

At the sixth, Arcline, body, life gets more subtle - the soul moves beyond direct communication and opens up to a sixth sense; intuition. Remembering its infinite connection, each soul must then listen and follow the guidance from within.

7. The Aura

Every seven years your body goes through a whole new cycle. Will you drop the baggage from your Aura and elevate yourself? Or continue to collect and weigh yourself down? When you create positive changes, you affect seven generations before and after you.

8. The Pranic Body

If you look at the figure of eight, you will see the infinite connection, which is found here – at the Pranic Body – through the breath; moment to moment; lifetime to lifetime; the cycle of life. Here the soul can learn to accept death and rebirth; can flow with life with each blessed breath. Or you can resist through fear and control and create illness.

9. The Subtle Body

The soul is almost home and so a deeper subtlety emerges; one that needs focus and acceptance of its true self, whilst also letting go of the end goal. Here, at The Subtle Body, you're presented with a choice to deep dive into mastery of truth or continue to circle the mystery of life.

10. The Radiant Body

The number 10, contains many of the qualities of the first, Soul Body (No.1), but the combination of this one with zero can offer either completion for the soul's journey or a removal of connection. The zero either enhances or nullifies the infinite connectedness of one – it's all or nothing now.

11. All-in-one

Here we see the relationship between the big I of the infinite and little I of the individual – The I and I as Rastafari's say. Is the soul now holding on to the individual form/will/ego, thereby making a double II and returning to the need of 2, or has true mergence been found?

#embodyyoursoulpurpose
@roisinallanakiernan

CALCULATING YOUR NUMBERS

We can understand and heal ourselves quicker when we understand that we are made up of ten bodies, of which some can be challenges (-) and others strengths (+).

Your Soul Number has to do with how you feel about yourself; Karma with how others see you; your Gift is your natural talent; your Destiny is a learnt talent; and Path your main challenge to gain overall fulfilment in this lifetime.

Use this simple Tantric Numerology calculation with your Date of Birth to explore your numbers. Any numerals, from the sections listed below, should be added together to form numbers between 1 and 11. Anything above 11, say 27, will need adding together, ie 2+7=9.

Please replace your Date of Birth with the numbers exampled below.

(-) SOUL NUMBER

(DAY YOUR WERE BORN, EG THE SIXTH - 6)

Your Soul Number is a challenge in this lifetime and is related to the roots on your Tree of Life. It's associated with your Father and the element of water and shows a challenge in the way you view yourself; a challenge that blocks you from connecting with your soul.

(-) KARMA NUMBER

(MONTH YOU WERE BORN, EG MAY - 5)

Your Karma Number is another challenge, related this time to the branches on your Tree of Life. It's connected with your peers (siblings and friends) and the element of fire. It shows how you are viewed by others and the difficulties this can raise.

(+) GIFT NUMBER 9+6=13 1+3=4

(DECADE YOU WERE BORN, EG '73 - 7+3 = 10)

Your Gift Number is a natural talent to use in this lifetime – a strength to harness. It relates to your Mother, the element of earth and the seeds on your Tree of Life. It's what you can offer to the world.

(+) DESTINY 1+9+9+6 = 25   2+5 = 7

(WHOLE YEAR, EG 1973 - 1+9+7+3 = 20 THEN 2+0 = 2)

Your Destiny Number shows a learnt and successful life strategy – another strength. It's the flower in your Tree of Life and is associated with air as well as your relationship with children.

(-) PATH 1+7+7+1+9+9+6 = 40 = 4

(ALL THE NUMBERS IN YOUR DATE OF BIRTH, EG 6+5+1+9+7+3 = 31 THEN 3+1 = 4)

Your Path Number offers the fruit in your Tree of Life. It's your relationship with a partner, is associated with the etheric elements and explains the action necessary to obtain overall fulfilment. This number, or body, is a challenge to assist you in gaining what you most wish for.

NB: This book's additional 'Tree of Life' knowledge descends from the wisdom of Shiv Charan Singh. Please see the Reference Page at the back of this book for further details.

(-) SOUL NUMBER
ROOTS (FATHER)

A challenge in the way you view yourself, which blocks you from connecting with your soul.

8

(-) KARMA NUMBER
BRANCHES (PEERS)

How you are viewed by others and the challenge this perception creates.

7

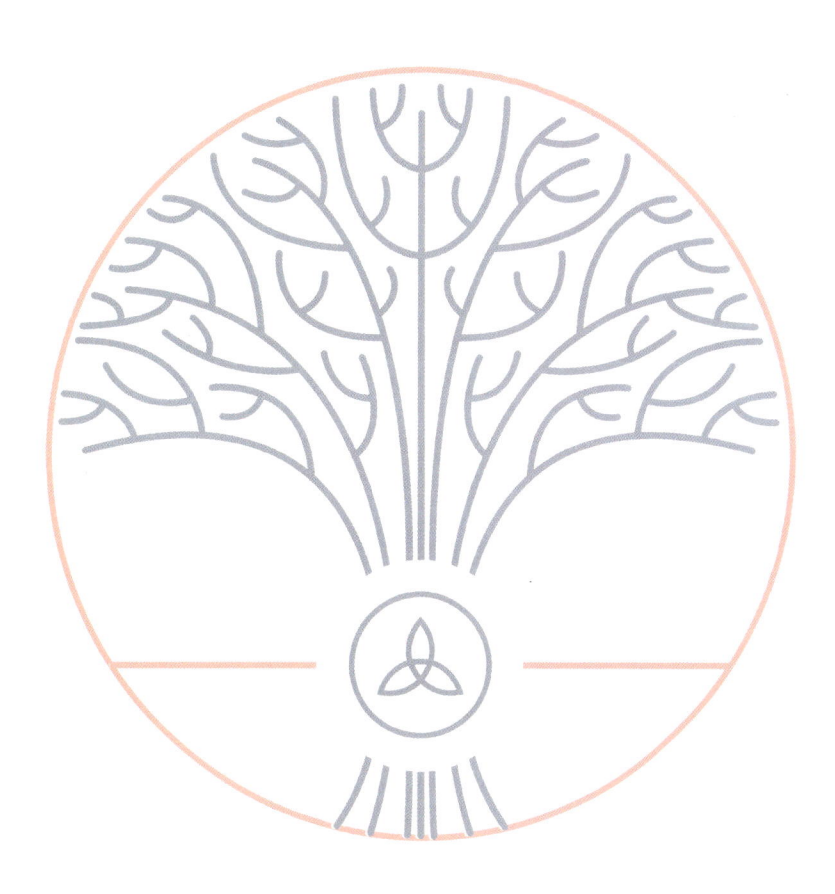

(+) GIFT NUMBER
SEED (MOTHER)

Your natural talent to use in this lifetime - what you can offer to the world.

4

(+) DESTINY NUMBER
FLOWER (CHILDREN)

Your learnt and successful life strategy.

7

PATH NUMBER - FRUIT (PARTNER)

The action necessary to obtain overall fulfilment.

4

#embodyyoursoulpurpose

@roisinallanakiernan

QUICK REFERENCE GUIDE

1. The Soul Body
HEAD OR HEART

Your infinite, all-connected essence – the true you, whispered through your heart's desires. When out of balance, you'll come more from your head than your heart.

2. The Protective (Negative) Mind
DIVISION OR UNITY

When out of balance, you'll be over-protective or negative, clinging on to people or situations as a method of control. Relationships (shown through the number 2) are important to this body.

3. The Projective (Positive) Mind
BALANCE INDIVIDUAL WILL WITH DIVINE WILL

A positive mental attitude helps us to achieve but then we must learn to trust and let go, with good humour, secure in the knowledge that all will work out as it should.

4. The Meditative (Neutral) Mind
BREATHE, THEN ACT

A meditative mind will 'tick-tock' between the pros and cons of each situation and find a place of neutrality between them.

5. The Physical Body
COMMUNICATION INCLUDES LISTENING

Five is the half way point to ten – the bridge, or communicative link; the teacher. Are you participating fully – receiving all messages and responding in service, for others and yourself?

6. The Arcline
WORRIER OR WARRIOR

Your halo, symbolised by a sword, which can be pointed at you (worry) or away from you (warrior). What you put out, or point towards yourself, all depends on you. Strengthen the subtleties of this body to alert and guide you with integrity.

7. The Aura
BAGGAGE OR ELEVATION

The magnetic field that surrounds your body can either trap you in patterns of reaction (your baggage) or bring awareness to protect and uplift in each moment with transparency.

8. The Pranic Body
THE INFINITE BREATH

Prana is the life force energy we take in through the breath, which flows in and out like the tide, coming and going, moment to moment. We can either flow with it or create resistance through fear and control, leading to illness.

9. The Subtle Body
MYSTERY OR MASTERY

Go deep into the core of you by staying put and focussing with discernment, discipline and patience. In this way you can choose mastery over your life, rather than circling the mystery.

10. The Radiant Body
ALL OR NOTHING

The combination of this 1 (Soul Body) with 0 can either offer infinite completion for the soul's journey or a removal of connection. You can either feel courageous or fearful; aspirational or unmotivated; confident or lacking self-esteem.

11. All-in-one
THE 'I AND I' RELATIONSHIP

Self-realisation through management of The Ten Bodies is incomplete without this additional relationship with The Divine. Without this relationship, you may seek reunion through another individual and return to the Number 2.

#embodyyoursoulpurpose
@roisinallanakiernan

A VISUAL REPRESENTATION

THE TEN BODIES

Take a moment to look at, read and then feel your way around the diagram on your right. It is my way of helping you understand and start to experience the intangible.

#embodyyoursoulpurpose

@roisinallanakiernan

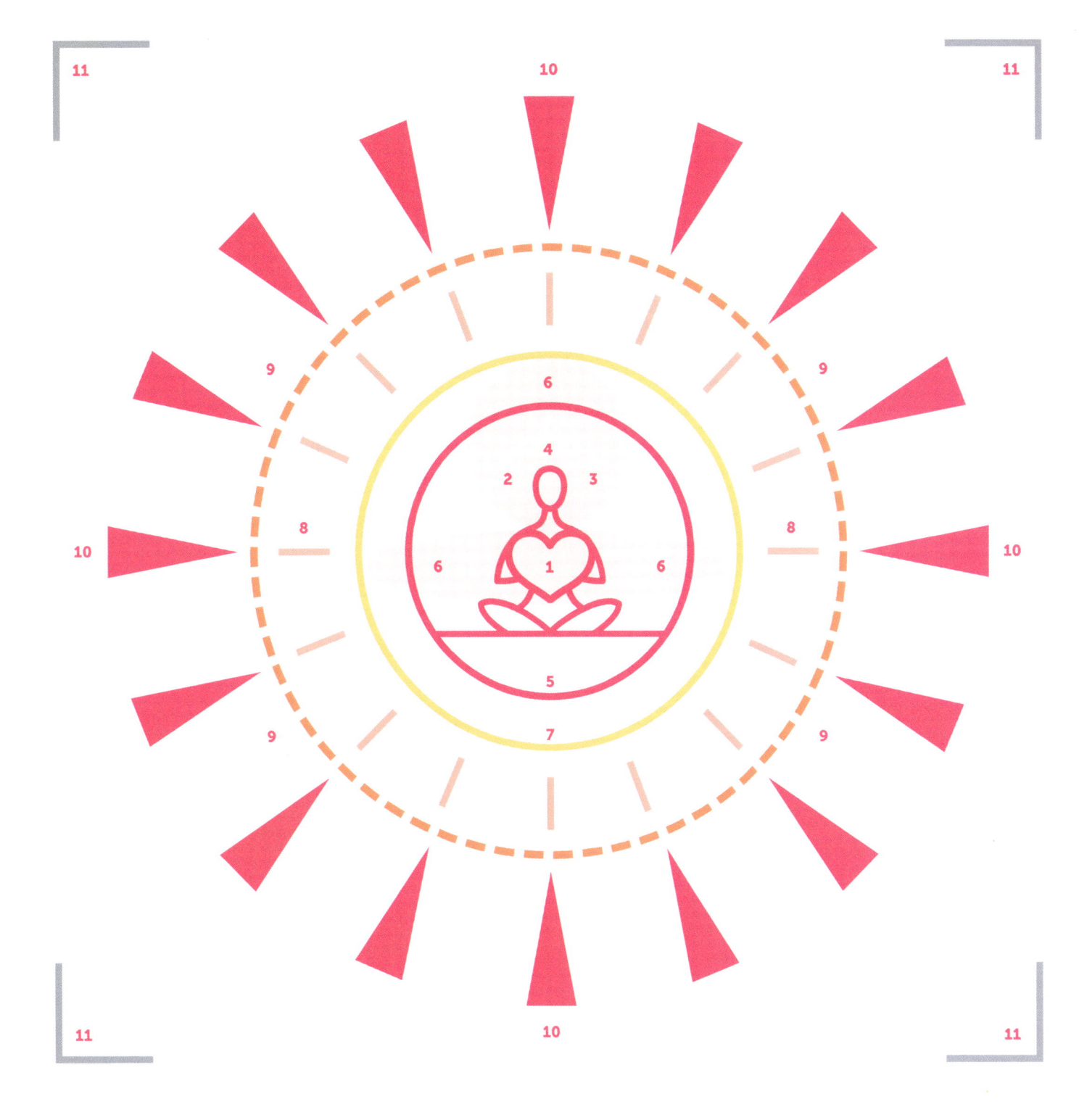

1. Soul Body
2. Protective Mind
3. Projective Mind
4. Meditative Mind
5. Physical Body
6. The Arcline
7. The Aura
8. The Pranic Body
9. The Subtle Body
10. The Radiant Body
11. All in One

TUNING IN & CLOSING THE SPACE

TUNING IN WITH THE ADI MANTRA

"Ong Namo Guru Dev Namo" X3
(I Bow To The Divine Within)

How do you feel about this statement? How does it feel to bow to the divine within you? Try not to judge or analyse just accept your response. To acknowledge that there's no separation between the outer and the inner divine creative power.

Ong means one, Namo is name or identity, Guru is the lesson when you go from darkness into the light and Dev is the great universal teacher. So, when you break it down in this way, the meaning could also be translated into – one name, the teacher within and the great universal teacher is one. You and the Divine (God, for want of another, less loaded, word) are one. I bow to the divine within.

Chant the Adi Mantra three times before beginning a class. You could also sing the mantra, and another beautiful way to connect with the depth of this meditation is through Celestial Communication (expressive movements to go with the mantra meditation).

Most of the mantras used in Kundalini Yoga are taken from the Sikh holy book, the Siri Guru Granth Sahib, and were created resonantly, rather than contextually like our modern languages. They are designed to hit the 84 keys or reflex points on the roof of your mouth that send signals to the hypothalamus (the regulatory gland in your brain, which then sends signals to secrete certain feelings within the body). These mantras are pure alchemy and will be explored further in this book.

You can also find videos of me explaining more about the Adi Mantra, chanting it and offering Celestial Communications with it, on my YouTube channel.

Accessed via my website – www.roisinallanakiernan.com

CLOSING THE SPACE

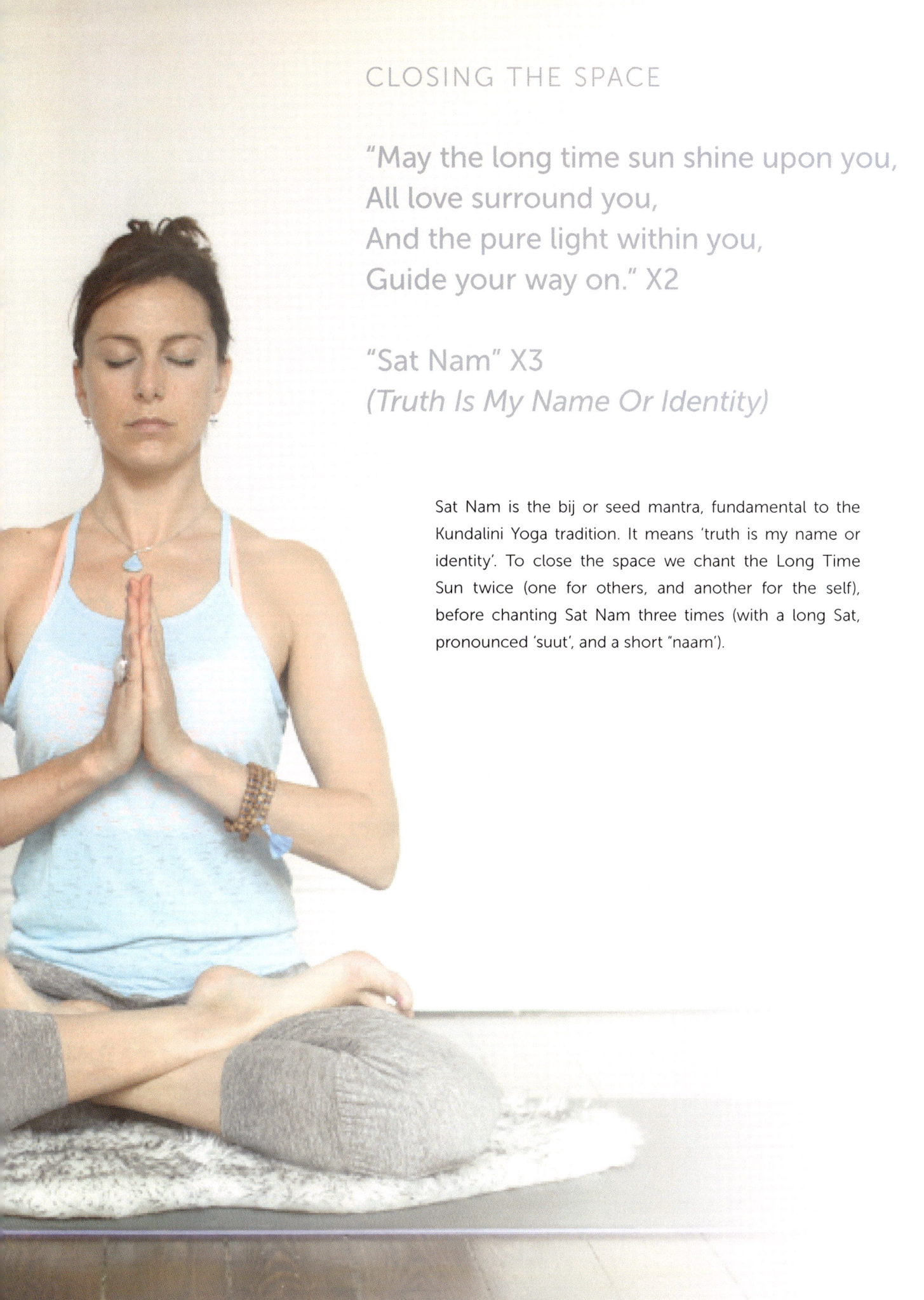

"May the long time sun shine upon you,
All love surround you,
And the pure light within you,
Guide your way on." X2

"Sat Nam" X3
(Truth Is My Name Or Identity)

Sat Nam is the bij or seed mantra, fundamental to the Kundalini Yoga tradition. It means 'truth is my name or identity'. To close the space we chant the Long Time Sun twice (one for others, and another for the self), before chanting Sat Nam three times (with a long Sat, pronounced 'suut', and a short "naam').

WARM UP EXERCISES

Most Kundalini Yoga classes will start by tuning in with the Adi Mantra and then move onto a few warm up exercises, carefully chosen depending on the kriya to follow.

If the kriya involves several hamstring or leg stretches then it is my preference to include a forward fold in the warm up. For more meditative kriya, I would add some spinal warm ups and head rolls - to get your energy moving.

Personally, my daily practise will often involve a few spinal warm ups to get my energy flowing before meditation. If I'm feeling a little sluggish or know my day will be fairly inactive, then I'll utilise a few sun salutations first too. Go with how your body feels.

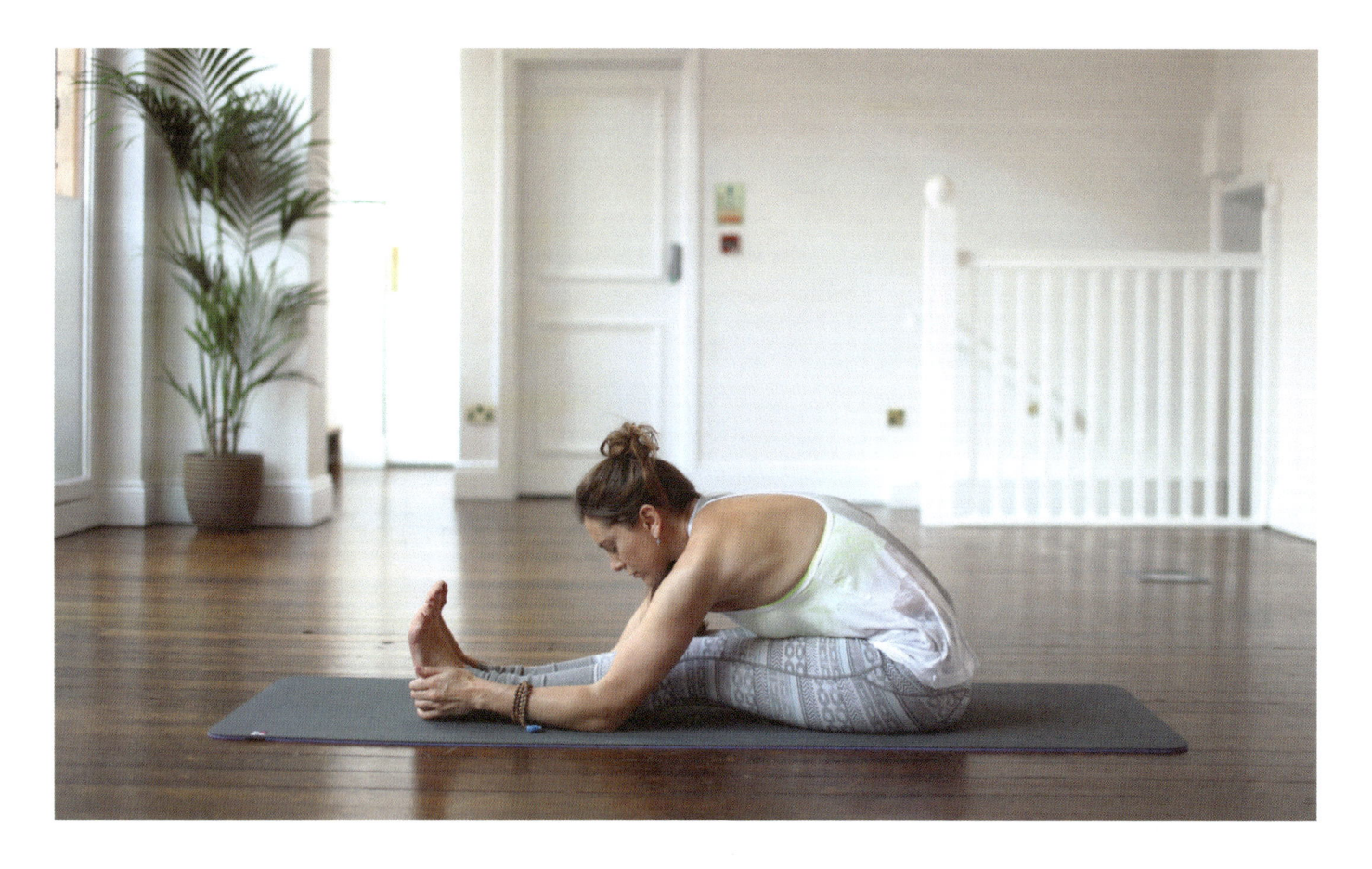

Forward Fold   1 Minute Minimum

Instructions: Sitting with your legs out straight and your feet pulled back towards you, inhale the arms up (palms facing) and then exhale over your legs. Hold this position with the spine straight. Roll your shoulders back, try to keep the chest open and lengthen through the spine with the breath.

Benefits: This stretches the sciatic (life) nerve, the hamstrings and lower back.

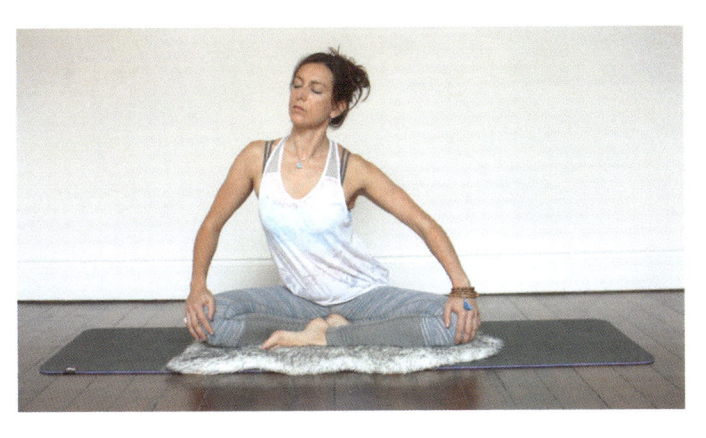

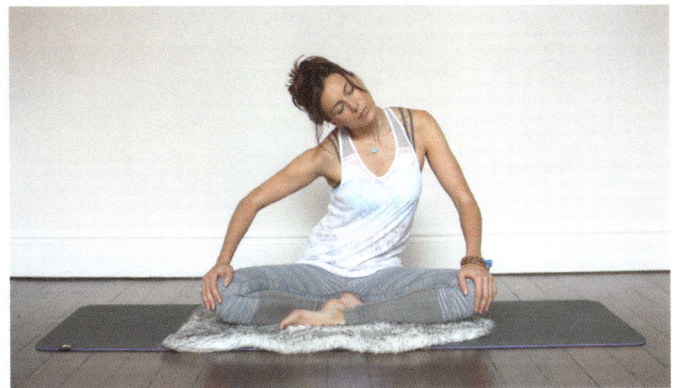

Torso Turns   Minimum 2 Minutes in Each Direction

Instructions: Sitting with a straight spine, inhale as you start rounding the torso forward, opening the chest and drawing the shoulders back, before exhaling as you round back. Imagine you're drawing circles around the body with your heart. Let your heart lead – the head follows; relax your neck.

Benefits: This warms the spine, eases through any tension and gently massages the inner organs.

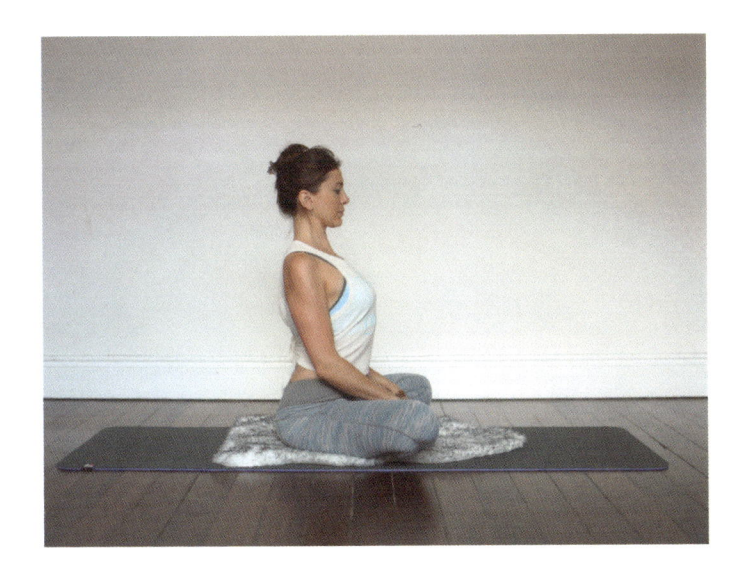

Spinal Flex   3 Minutes

Instructions: Sitting tall with the legs crossed, take hold of your shins and, keeping the head in line with the base of your spine, inhale as you arch your torso forward (opening chest and shoulders) and exhale as you round back. The head doesn't move.

Benefits: This works to bring strength and flexibility to the lower back. After 3 minutes, the brain wave patterns change, making you more calm.

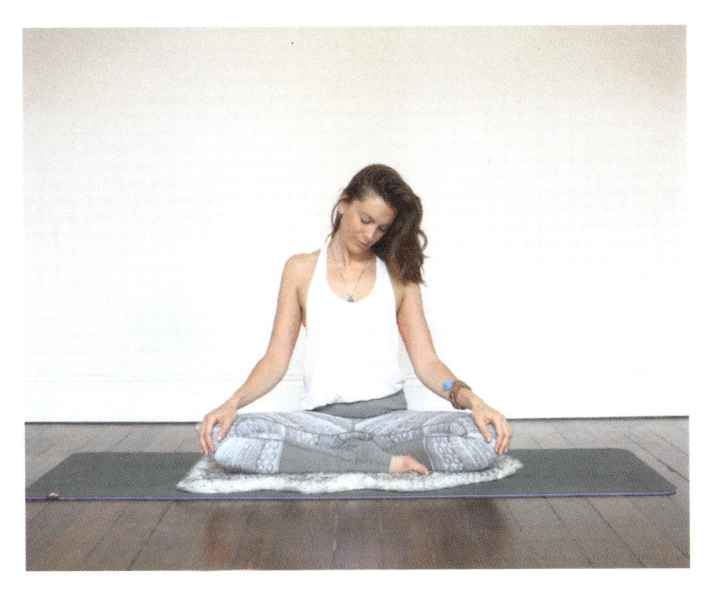

Head & Shoulder Rolls

7-8 Rolls in Each Direction

Instructions: Sitting with hands on your knees, begin rolling the shoulders forwards and up as you inhale and back around as you exhale. Do these a few times before going the other way, then move to the neck - inhaling as you round forwards and down and exhaling as you round back.

Benefits: This opens the blood flow to the head, releases any tension in the neck and shoulders and rejuvenates the brain.

THE SUN SALUTATION

The Sun Salutation - Surya Namaskara A - offers a great all-round warm up. I find this especially useful when using kriyas that are fairly stationary, this is because the Sun Salutation gets the circulation going and gives most body parts a good old stretch.

Move with the breath, starting on an inhale as your reach up and then exhale or inhale subsequently with each movement. You might also like to start slow and hold each position for a few breaths, building up speed with each round. I would suggest five as the minimum number of cycles.

As we reach to the Heavens from our hearts, The Sun Salutation draws active solar energy down into the body. Then, as we bow down, we honour the Earth and our connection to it before circulating this energy throughout our system and bowing once more, rising to draw in that solar energy and finishing in the heart. In this way, The Sun Salutation offers a complete cycle of connection – between our body, mind and breath as well as the Earth, ourselves and Heaven. Indeed, the sun could well be representative of the light or the Divine and the bowing down to it as an opportunity to cleanse our bodies and minds from darkness.

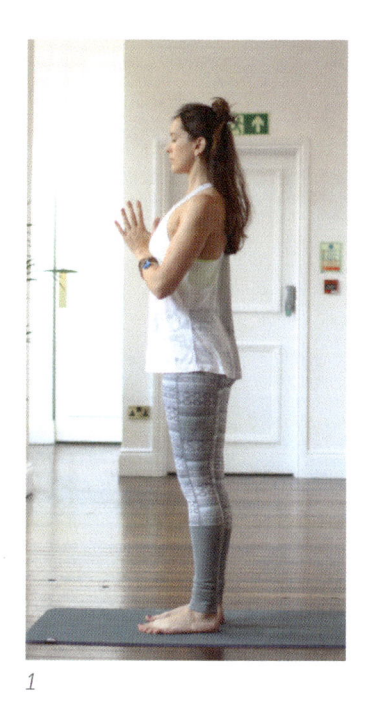

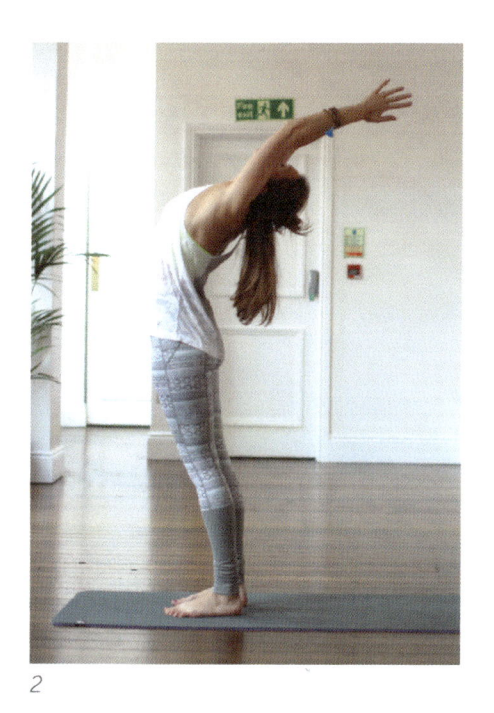

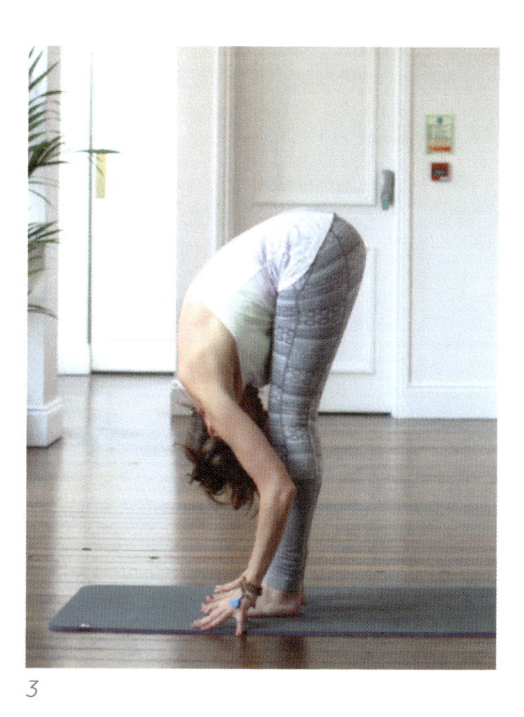

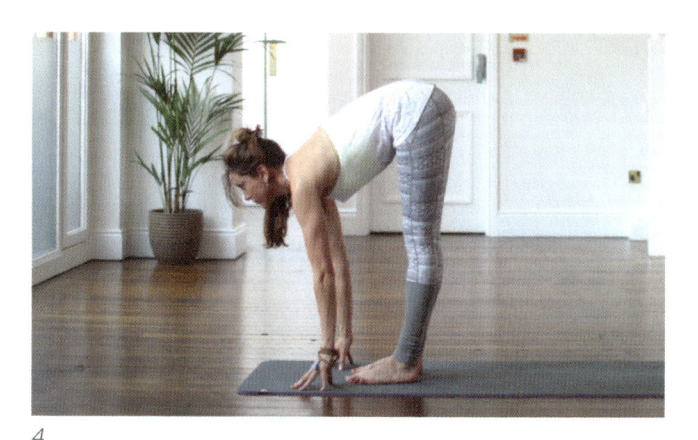

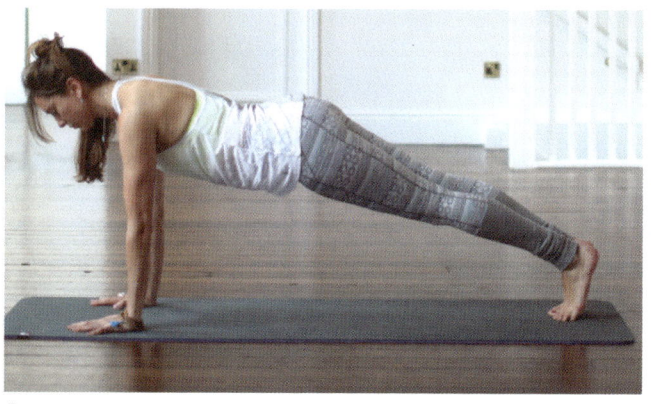

1

2

3

4

5

6

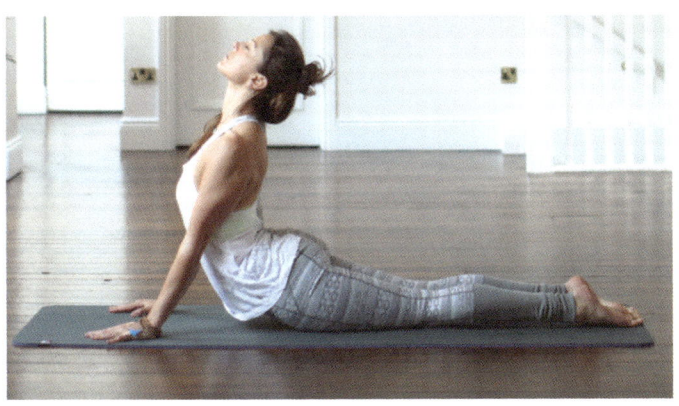

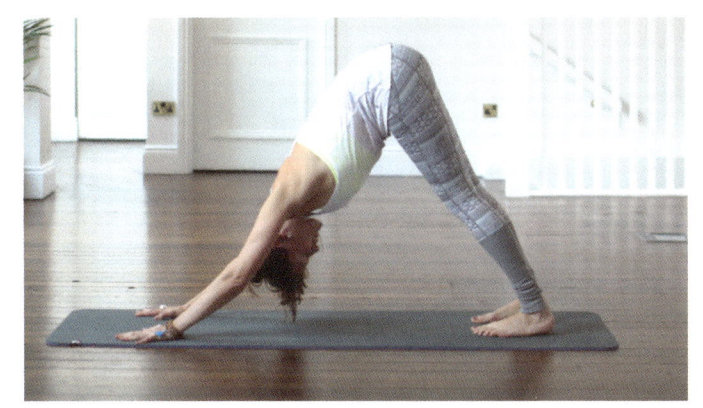

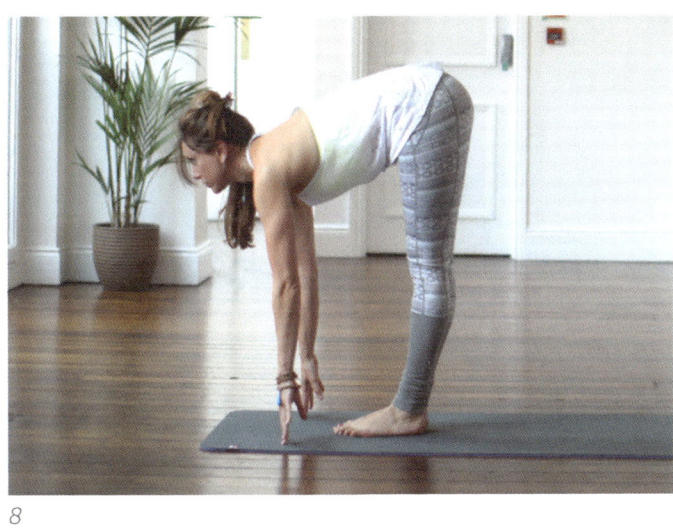

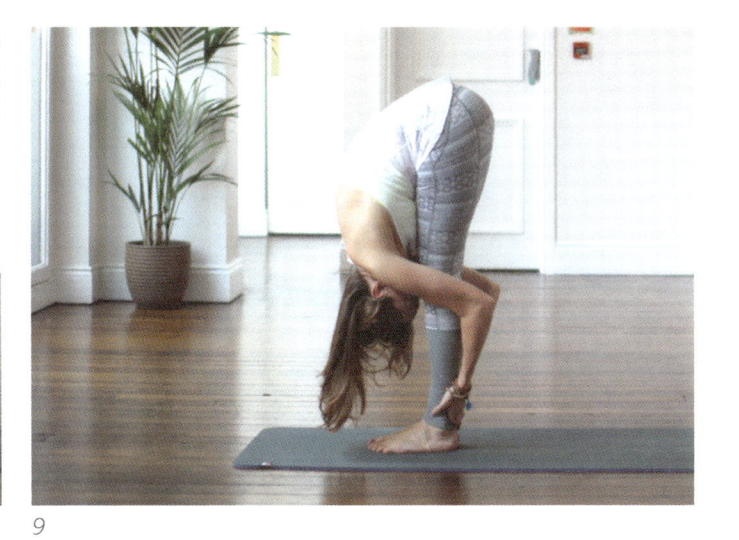

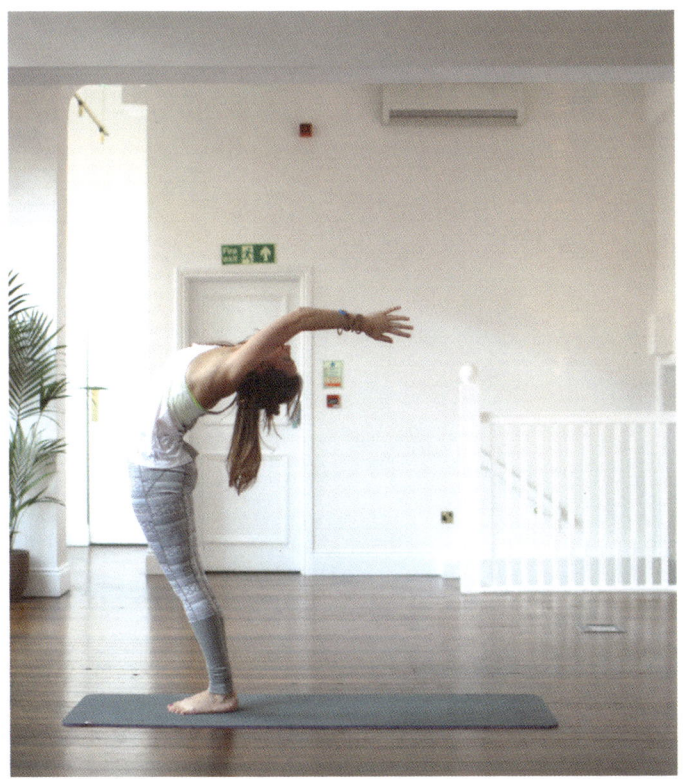

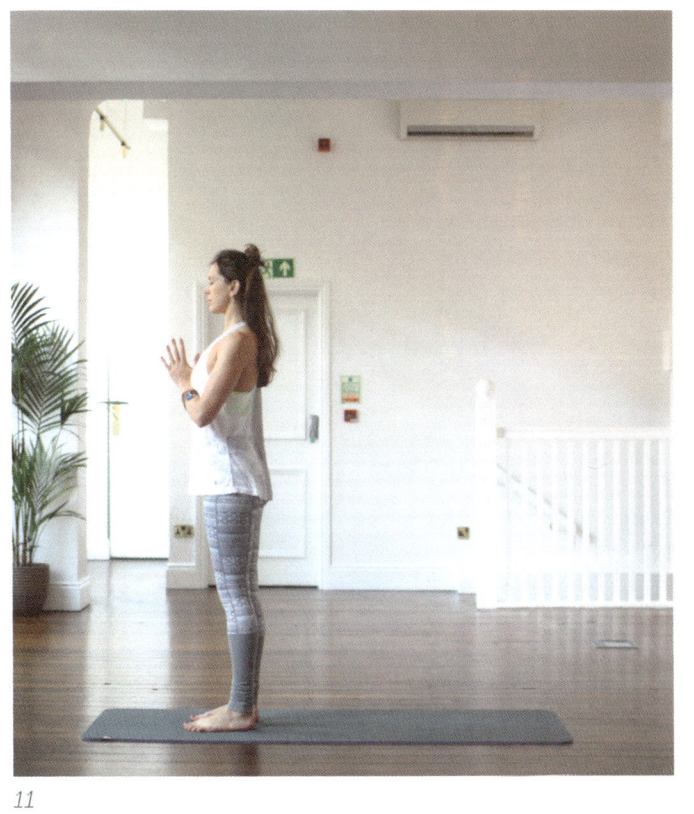

7

8

9

10

11

25

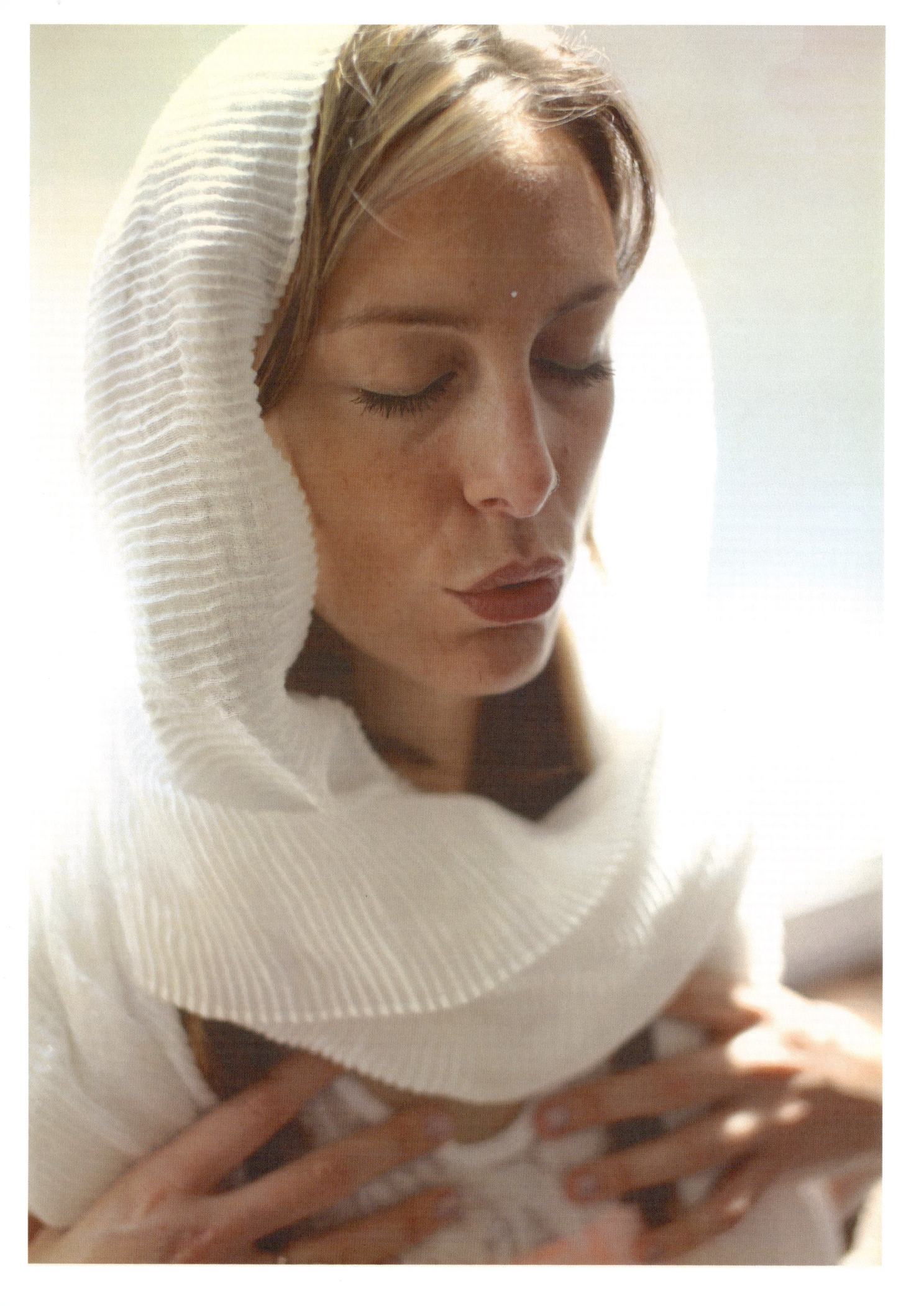

1

THE SOUL BODY

HEAD OR HEART

The key to being a spiritual being is to come from your heart. The person who has a conflict with their first spiritual body will come more from their head than from their heart.

#embodyyoursoulpurpose
@roisinallanakiernan

THE SOUL BODY
HEAD OR HEART

The Soul Body often has a battle going on - between your head and heart or ego and intuition. By negating your feelings (your heart's desires and intuition) you deny your true needs. By over-valuing intellect you lose sight of your true, soul self.

You know you best though – you have only to listen. Even the greatest so-called Guru cannot tell you about you – they simply guide you back to your wisdom, to your true, soul self. They are your torchbearers, summoned by you to guide you from darkness to light – the very meaning, in fact, of Guru. Your soul even has a Personal Assistant - the Subtle Body, which records everything you do, relaying notes on topics that need work and supporting you through multiple journeys.

The problem is that your intellect is often in competition with your soul – distracting, confusing and striving to keep you in a false, protective bubble of individualism. You might, for instance, be in a job, relationship or lifestyle which you're clinging to through fear, even though you know it's not serving you. Even though, underneath that self-enslaved armour is a wisdom, trust and support network that needs no protection.

The Soul Body doesn't work alone though. Just as 1 is part of 10, the Soul Body is part of Ten Bodies and we are all simultaneously individuals that are part of one universal whole. Too strong an individual will and you'll be looking after No.1 – your soul will not truly be in union with its universal, collective state. Alternatively, with humility, a strong soul can step forward as the voice for the group.

A suppressed soul will force its way to the surface too, often sabotaging the very blocks of oppression that have denied its natural expression. Losing a job, being bed-ridden or splitting up with a partner can be happening for you, rather than to you - working like cosmic order - you have only to read the signs.

With The Soul Body balanced we trust and are compassionate (about ourselves and others). We give and receive in equal measure. We can stand strong in ourselves yet feel others too, without getting caught up in their drama. We are in love with life and living in love.

When we follow our feelings, our heart/inner soul self, we live in love - the natural seat of the soul. Because, by doing what we love and sharing that we create a world based on truth, on authenticity, because in every moment we're following what feels right, rather than acting or doing in a way that isn't true. That doesn't mean throwing intelligence away but using it to work our true self, our soul's desire, whilst being mindful and patient about our own and others' journeys and remembering that we are all imperfectly perfect and rolling through our own endless journeys, as one and the same.

Trust yourself. Follow your bliss and you'll be more fulfilled, more rich, more wealthy in a very healthy kind of way.

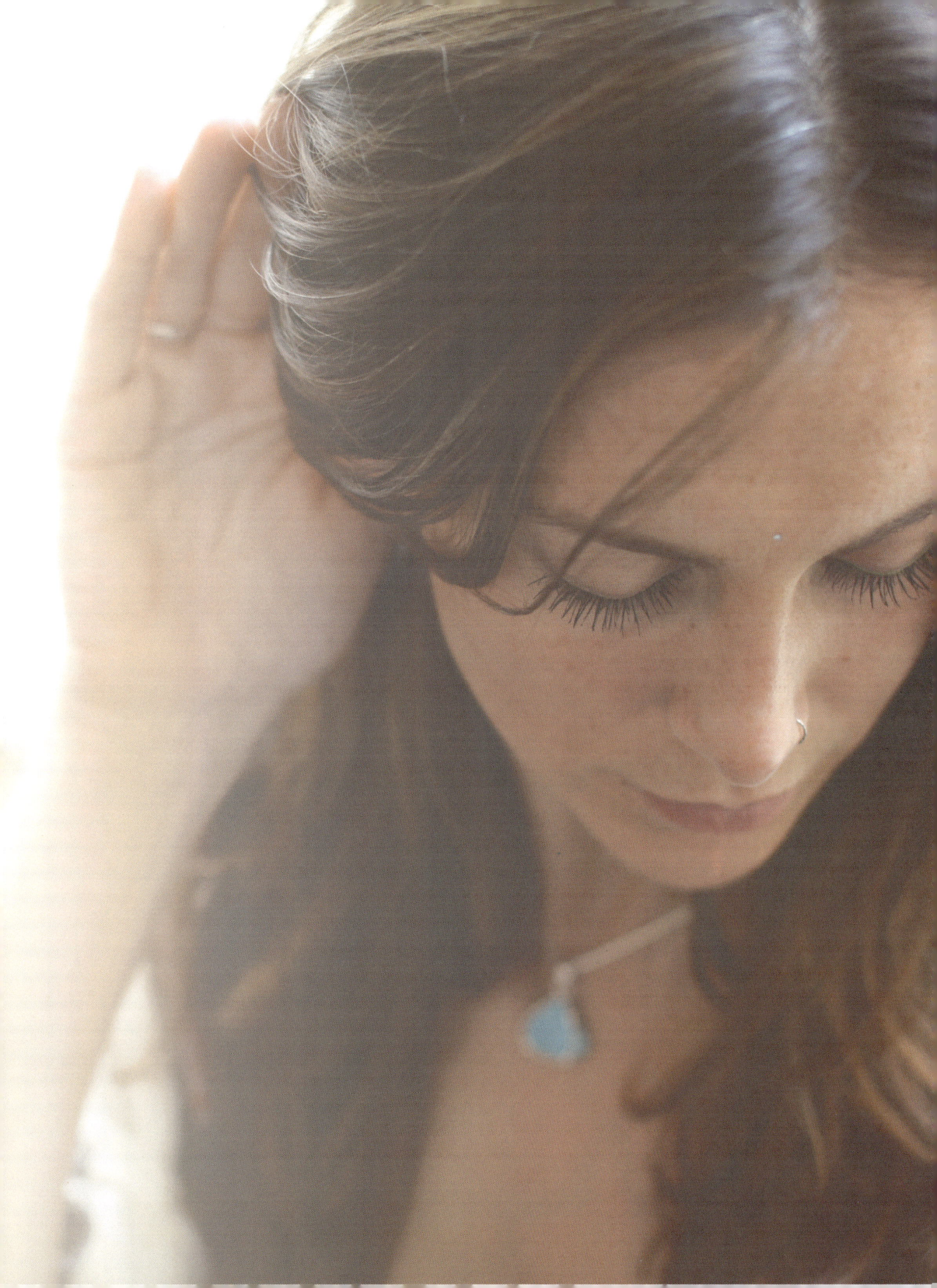

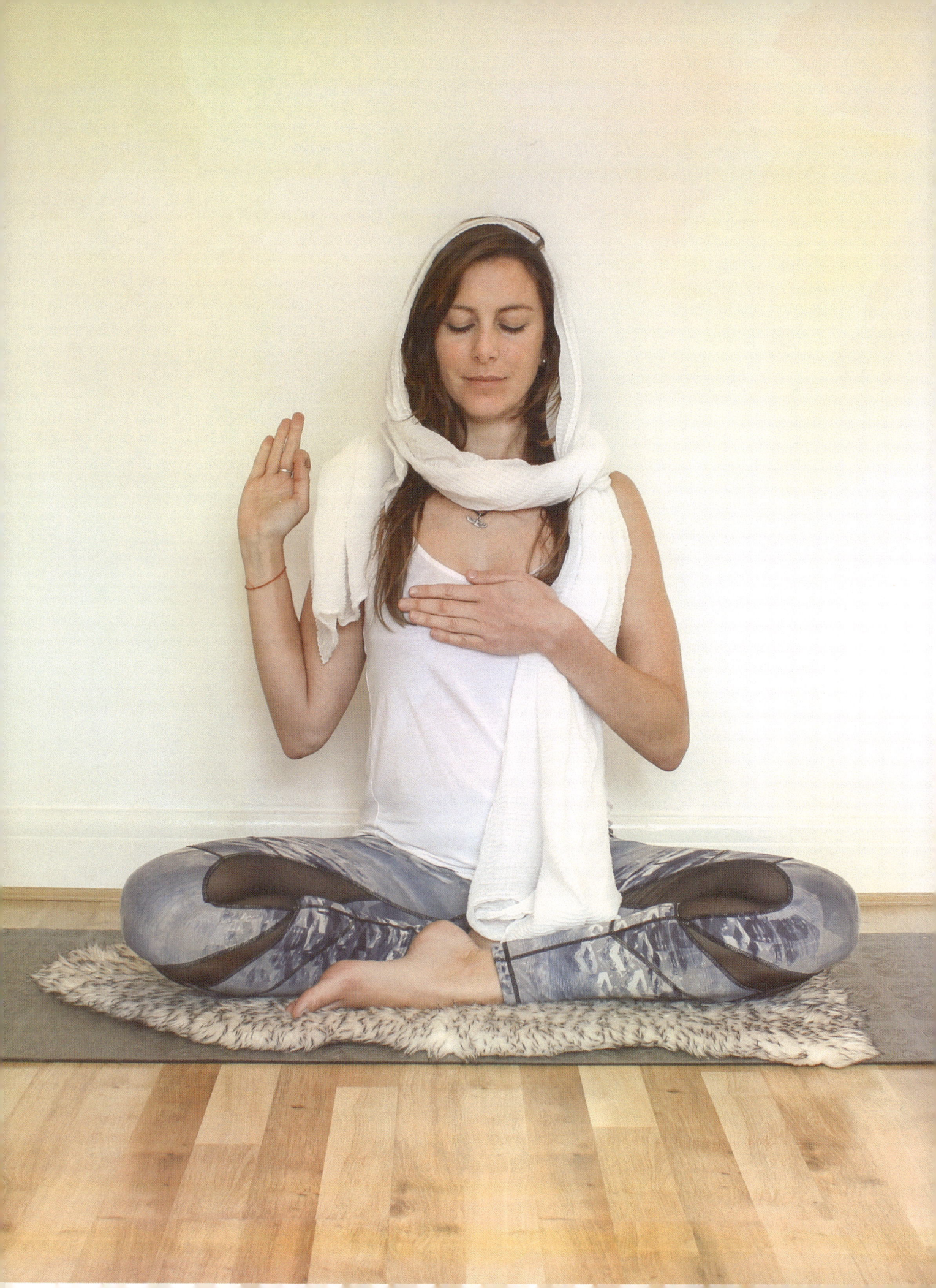

PRANAYAMA
MEDITATION FOR A CALM HEART

POSITION

Sit comfortably with your spine straight. The eyes may be closed or nine tenths closed looking straight ahead.

Place the left hand on the chest at the Heart Centre. The palm is flat against the chest and the fingers are parallel to the ground, pointing to the right. Make Gyan Mudra with the right hand (touch the tip of the index finger with the tip of the thumb) and raise it up to face out from the right shoulder, as if giving a pledge. The elbow is relaxed by your side.

BREATH

Inhale slowly and deeply through both nostrils, suspend the breath in and raise the chest. Retain this breath and position for as long as possible then exhale smoothly, gradually, and completely. When the breath is totally out, lock the breath out for as long as possible.

DURATION

Continue this pattern of long, deep breathing for 3-31 minutes.

TO END

Inhale and exhale strongly 3 times then relax.

COMMENTS

The entire posture in this meditation is designed to make you feel calm.

The left palm (feminine side) is placed at the natural home of prana (the breath/subtle life force energy), creating a deep stillness at that point. The right hand, which throws you into action and analysis (masculine) is placed in a receptive, relaxed mudra (energy seal) and put in the position of peace.

Emotionally, this meditation offers clarity to your relationships, both with yourself and others. Any time you feel upset, or out of balance in a situation, try this meditation for 3 to 15 minutes before deciding how to act. Then act with your full heart.

Physically, this meditation strengthens the lungs and heart.

It is perfect for beginners, as it opens awareness of the breath and conditions the lungs.

In a class try it for 3 minutes. If you have more time, try it for three periods of 3 minutes each, with 1 minute of rest between them, for a total of 11 minutes. For an advanced practice of concentration and rejuvenation, build the meditation up to 31 minutes.

#embodyyoursoulpurpose
@roisinallanakiernan

KRIYA 1

FOR BALANCING HEAD AND HEART

This set opens, balances and clears the Heart Chakra (heart-based energy centre). Remember, that a person who is not in touch with their Soul Body, will come more from their head than their heart – this set can re-balance that. On a physical level, the exercises will strengthen the heart, lungs, shoulders and chest as well as promoting better circulation and detoxifying the body. It also works to soften one's character, dropping the person into the heart; a space of love, compassion and forgiveness.

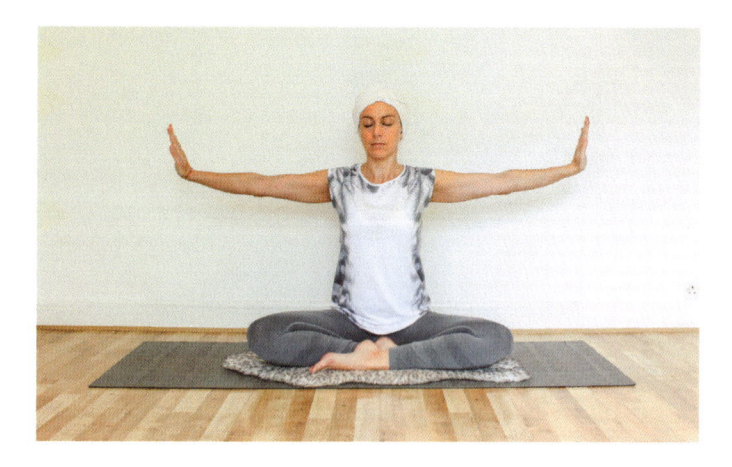

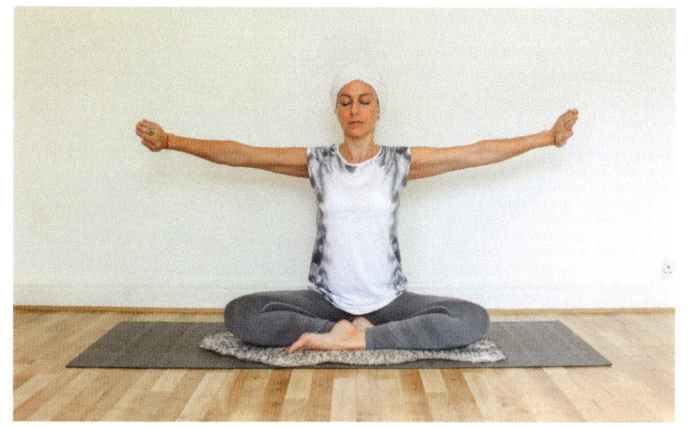

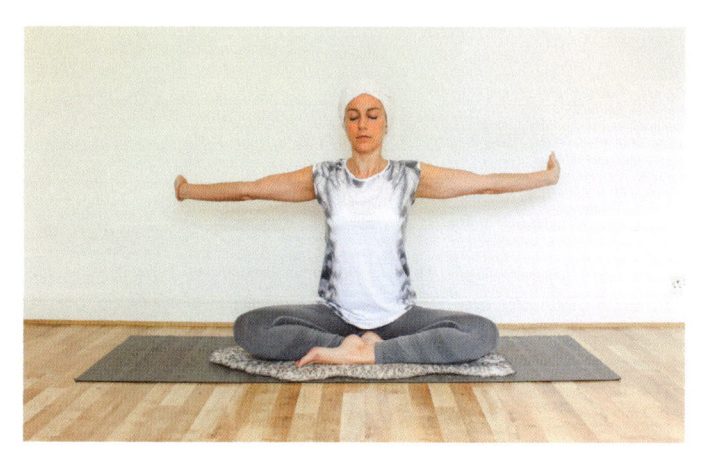

1. Changing The Chemistry Of The Brain
6-7 Minutes

Instructions: Sit crossed legged with a straight spine and your arms straight out to the sides with the hands bent up at the wrists, palms facing out and fingers up.

The movement is in four parts; starting with the beginning position (1), then rotating the hands at the wrists so the fingers point forward (2), before rotating back to the original position (3), and then rotating the wrists so the fingers point straight backwards (4).

Inhale when your fingers point upwards and exhale each time they rotate forwards or backwards.

Move in a rhythm of one full cycle per 4 seconds. Keep the arms straight.

Benefits: Works to clarify the mental processes. It also strengthens the arms, chest, upper back and shoulders.

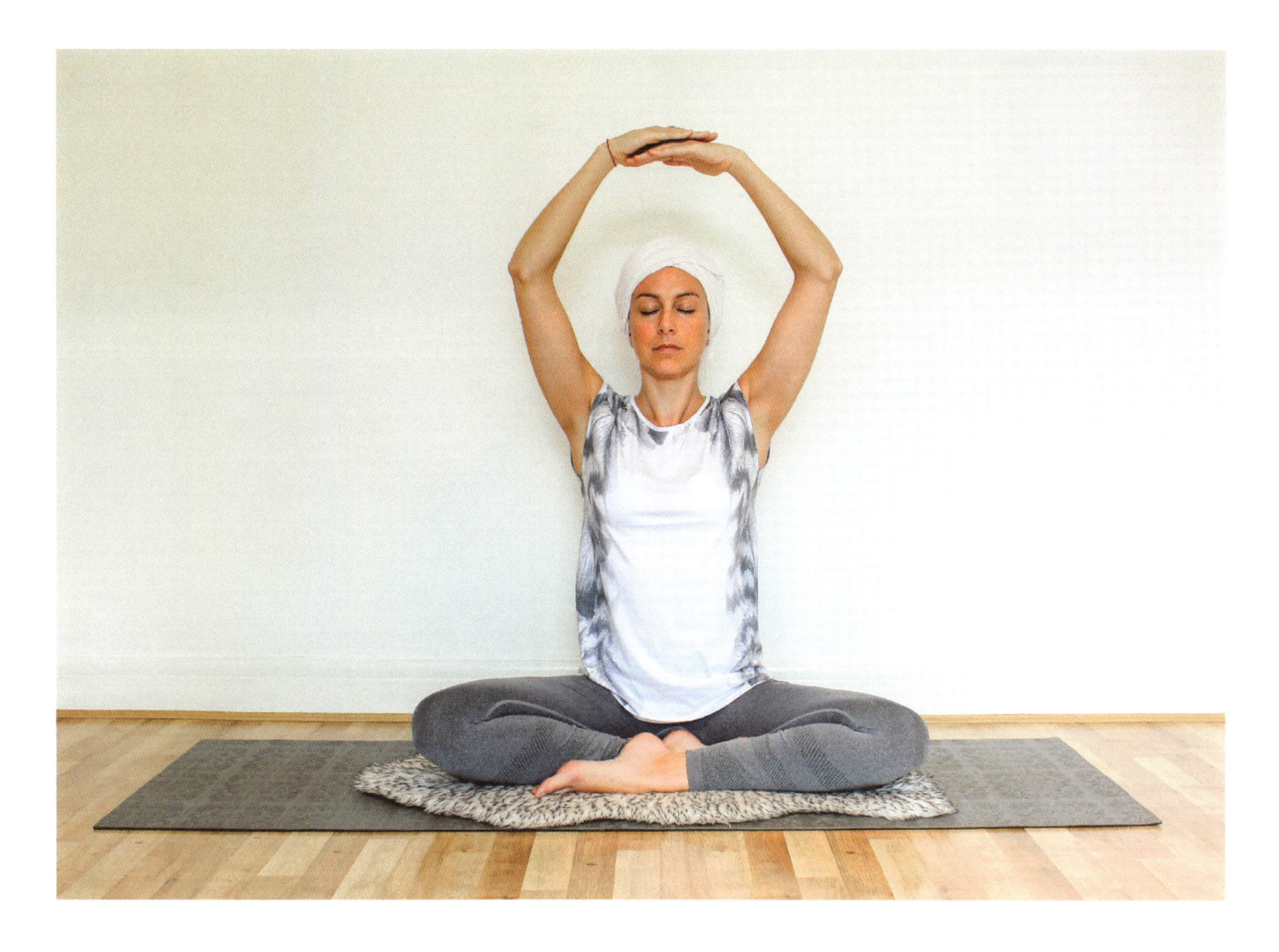

2. Lifting Arms Overhead
1-2 Minutes

Instructions: Still sitting, extend the arms straight out to the sides, palms facing out, then inhale the arms into an arc (palms crossing) slightly in front of the top of the head, before exhaling to the start position. Then, when you inhale the arms up into an arc again, bring the hands (palms crossing) slightly behind the top of the head, and again exhale back to the start position. Continue in this way, inhaling up (alternating between in front of and behind the head), and exhaling to the start position.

Continue the motion powerfully and always keep the arms parallel to the floor in the start position.

Benefits: Strengthens the arms, shoulders, chest and upper back. As well as working the brain.

3. Adding Crow Squats
3-4 Minutes

Instructions: Stand up and add crow squats to the arm movements of exercise 2 – inhaling up into the start position and exhaling down into Crow Squat with the alternating arm positions.

Crow Pose is a crouching position with the knees drawn into the chest and the soles of the feet flat on the floor.

Continue at a speed of 1 second per movement.

Benefits: This brings greater coordination with the legs, plus strengthens the lower half of the body, as well as the arms, chest, upper back and shoulders.

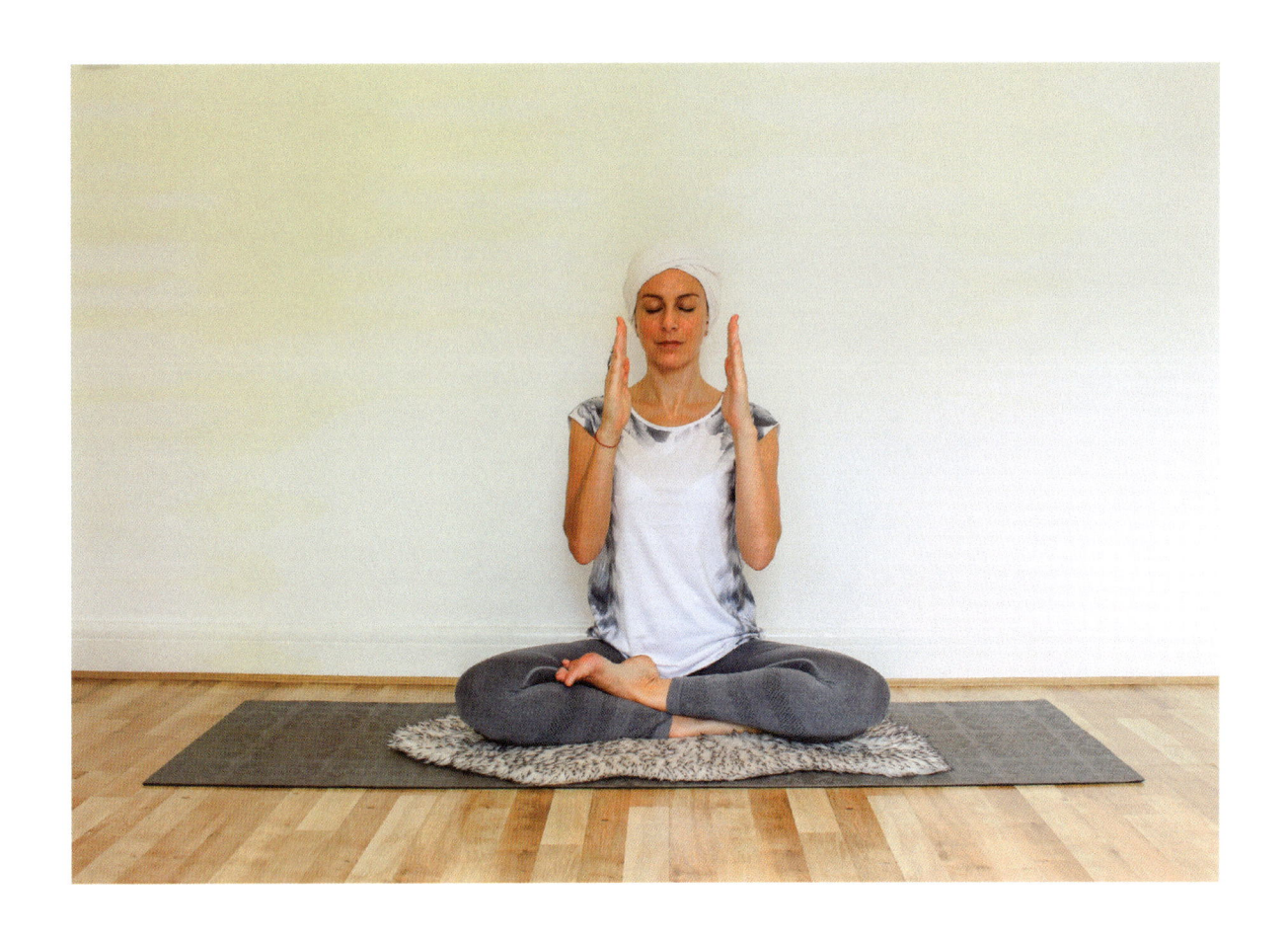

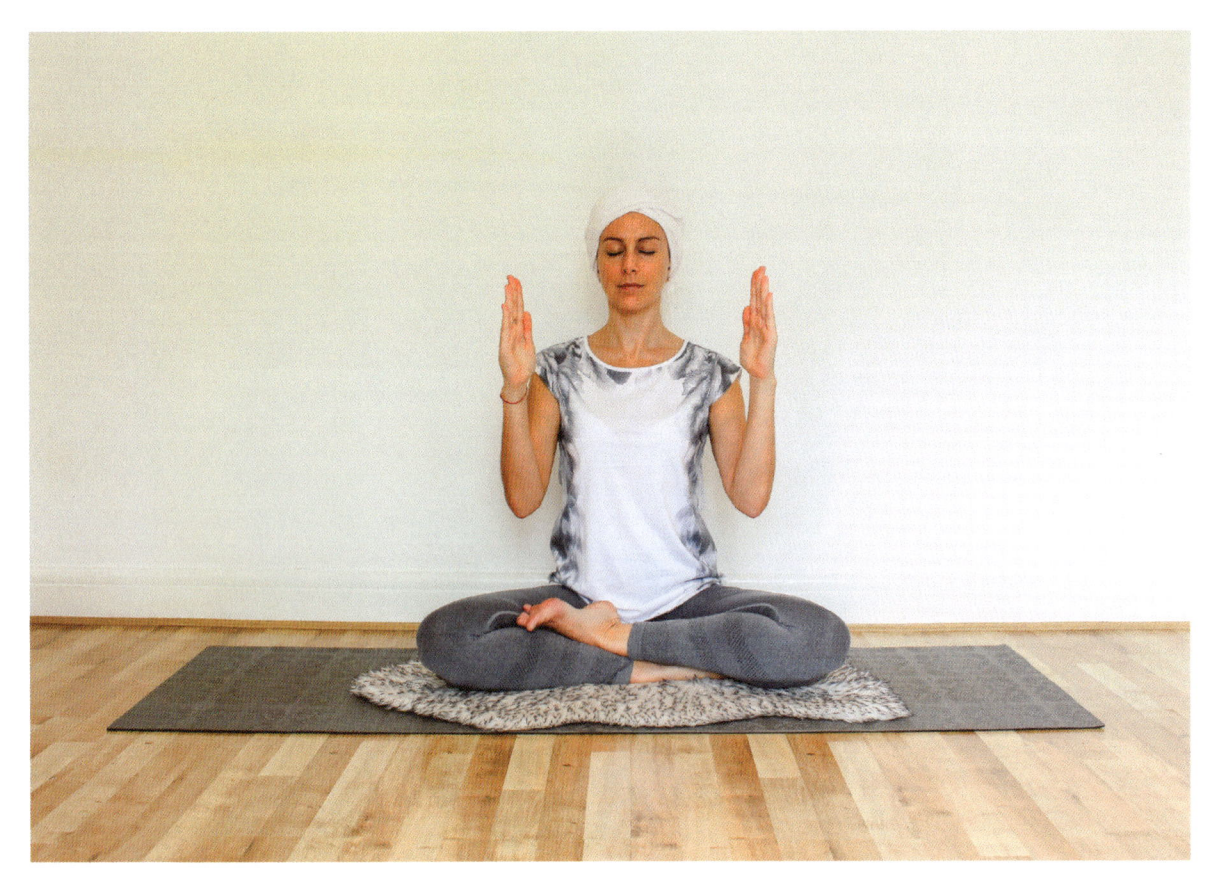

KRIYA 2

MEDITATION TO OPEN THE LOCK OF THE HEART AND INCREASE THE POWER OF THE INFINITE WITHIN

11 Minutes

Instructions: Sit crossed legged with a tall spine and a light neck lock (Jalandhar Bandha).

Bring the hands about 6-8 inches in front of your face, palms flat and facing one another, fingers pointing towards the ceiling, and with about 6-8 inches between the palms. Elbows are relaxed down.

With a very fast, powerful jerk stretch the hands out until there is about 36 inches between them and abruptly stop them. Then, instantly, the hands will recoil back to the first position in front of the body.

The stopping process will be so abrupt, done with such a powerful force, that you'll find the hands, chest, shoulders, and head jerking back and forth a little bit.

Mantra: Use the 'Tantric Har' recording to move with.

Har

Use the rhythm of the recording Tantric Har and stretch the arms back with a jerk on each Har, which means We or God/The Divine. Do not sing aloud.

To End: Inhale and suspend the breath, but keep on doing the motion on the held breath for 15 seconds. Exhale. Inhale again and continue the motion for 10 seconds. Exhale. Inhale deeply, continue, holding for 5 seconds. Relax.

Benefits: The navel area, the Third Chakra, is sometimes referred to as the agan granthi – the place from which all fire-related activities spring; food, digestion, breath, etc. When this center is locked, your ribcage can become out of place. Then the diaphragm doesn't act right, and you lose one third of your life force. This meditation releases this lock and will open up the power of the Infinite within you.

Shock your subtle nervous system on the sound of Har, and jolt your heart open.

MEDITATION

BALANCING MIND AND HEART UNTO INFINITY

POSITION

Sit with a straight spine and bring your hands onto your chest with thumbs tucked into armpits. Rest your palms and fingers against the chest. Elbows relax by the sides. Eyes are nine tenths closed.

BREATH

Pucker the lips and inhale deeply through the mouth with a whistle. Listen to the sound of this whistling inhale as you mentally say 'So'.

Then exhale through the nose as you listen to the breath and mentally say 'Hung'.

So Hung means, 'I Am Infinity'.

MANTRA

So Hung

DURATION

11 minutes

COMMENTS

It is through the understanding that comes from the heart – of Universal Consciousness; of unity – that the mind can realise the concept that Infinity is within.

#embodyyoursoulpurpose
@roisinallanakiernan

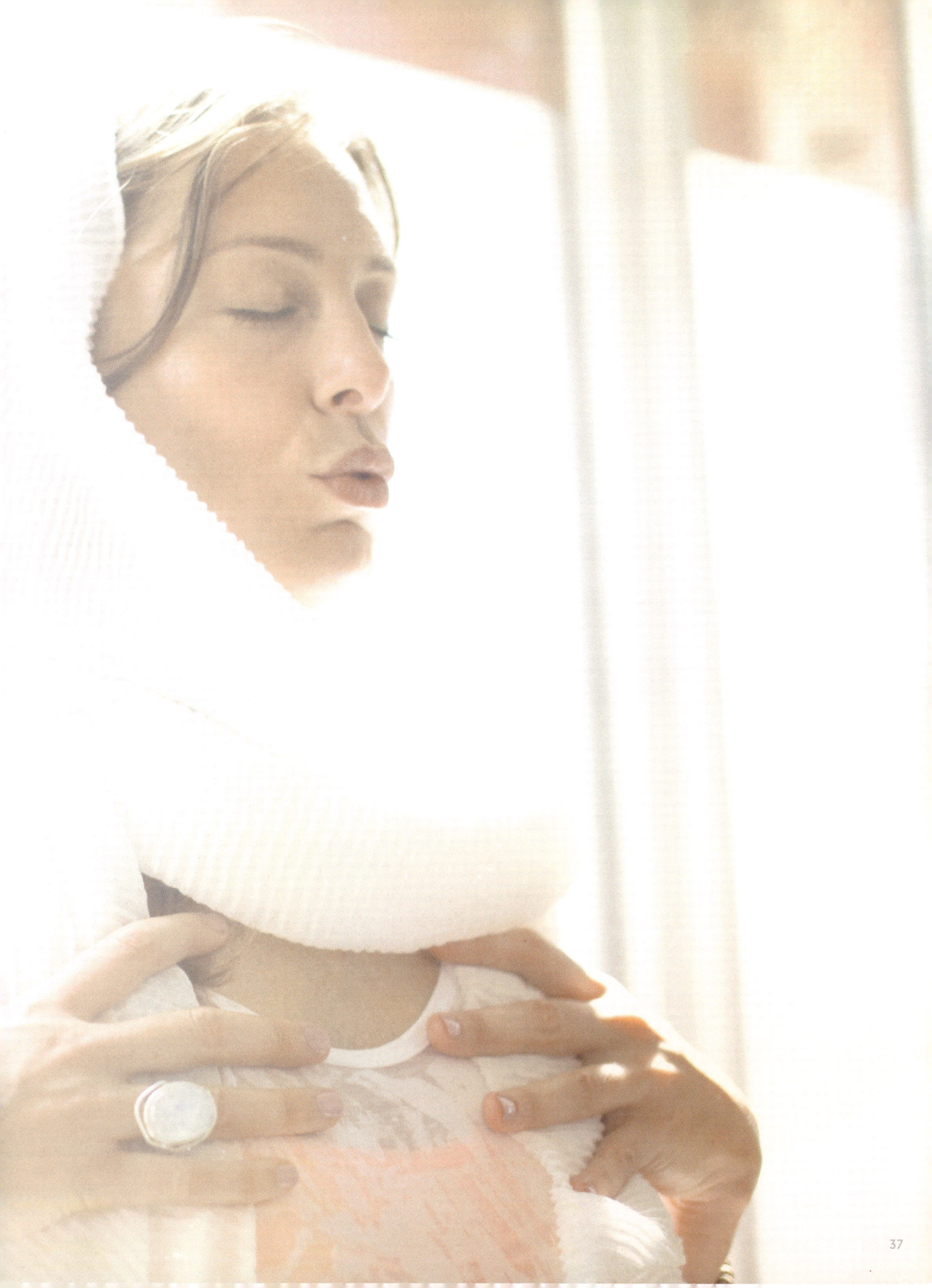

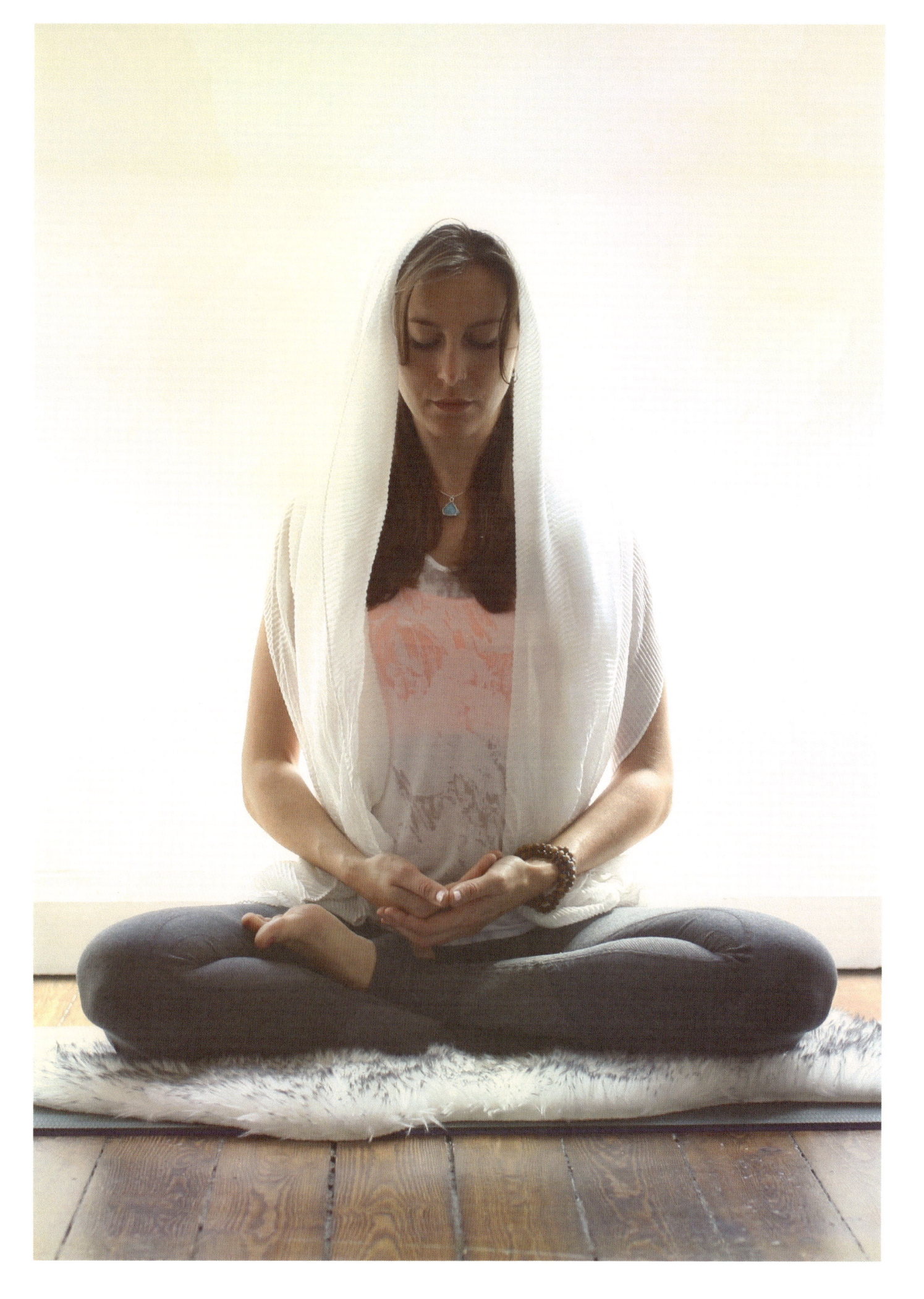

②

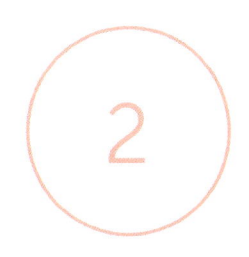

THE PROTECTIVE (NEGATIVE) MIND

DIVISION OR UNITY

When out of balance, you'll be over-protective or negative, clinging on to people or situations as a method of control. Relationships (shown through the number 2) are important to this body.

#embodyyoursoulpurpose
@roisinallanakiernan

THE PROTECTIVE (NEGATIVE) MIND
DIVISION OR UNITY

The second, Protective (or Negative) Body, takes us into division (it's a step away from the universal whole of the Soul Body position at 1). The second body also offers an opportunity to bring whole units (two whole people) together in a step towards unity. Two, therefore, is about relationships - about reflection, emotion and movement - in correlation with its element of water.

When your soul split from the universal into physical form an immediate 'longing to belong' was created. And this journey (back to belonging) is taking place through the physical and, therefore, through relationship. You draw in people and scenarios necessary for your soul's journey back to the Infinite.

Your soul yearns to return to its universal, Infinite form and this division creates a negative state with needs that pull you into relationships (an attempt to have your needs met by another). You might be looking for a relationship to feel secure, loved or supported, which are all aspects of a positive relationship but they must also be found in yourself. In order to meet another as a whole individual you must first fall in love with yourself – learn to feel, recognise and then meet your own needs.

All problems in relationship will be reflecting back your needs. The way in which people treat you will be a mirror for how you feel about yourself. How is your own self-worth? You set the bar for how people treat you.

Often your needs can be traced back to childhood or another incident in the past which made you feel like you had to protect yourself (the task of the Negative Mind). Any future scenarios that then trigger the hurt feeling from before (albeit subconsciously) can make you react and will continue to trigger you until you heal the underlying pain.

Ignored needs overflow from the subconscious as toxic thoughts, which then pour out in unhealthy actions. This feeling of emptiness, of disconnection (from our soul's 'longing to belong'), can lead to addictions too – food, drugs, drink, sex, people – all of which are used to 'fill the void'. You could also become attached to your needs – to the drama – forgetting that these needs are actually an opportunity to learn and grow and, therefore, return to our soul's Infinite connection.

All illness begins in the Protective Mind. When you're out of synch with your soul – when you refuse to acknowledge and work through the lessons being offered, or become attached to a singular need – then blockages will form in your body. Your energy can either flow in a healthy way – moving through needs and lessons - or it can become stagnant and unhealthy.

Loyalty is a more positive aspect of The Protective Mind, providing the opportunity to discipline yourself with habits such as meditation, which will help you see your destructive patterns and offer the space needed to make changes, therefore aiding your soul's growth. This same loyalty can, of course, keep you stuck in negative patterns too.

41

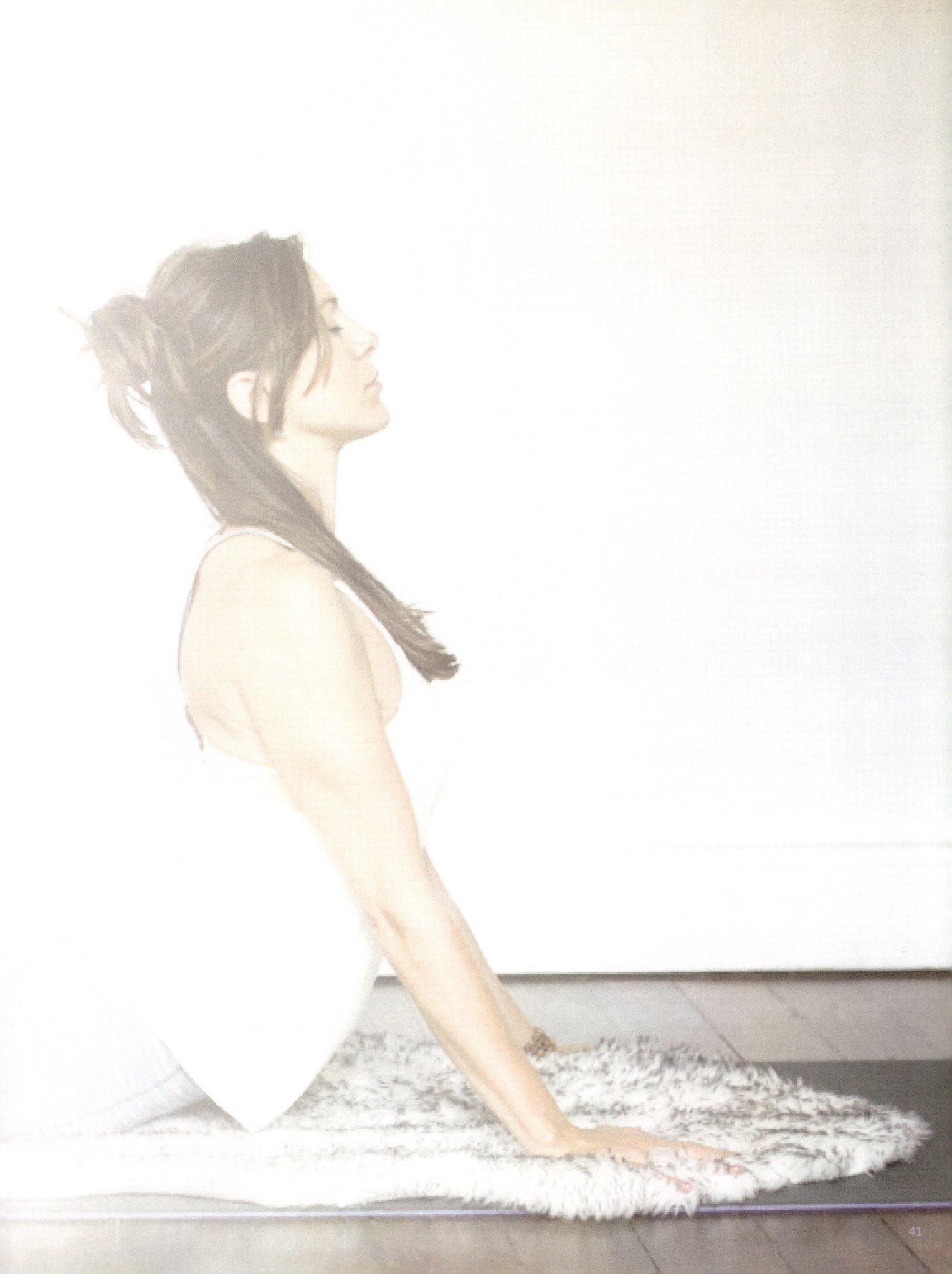

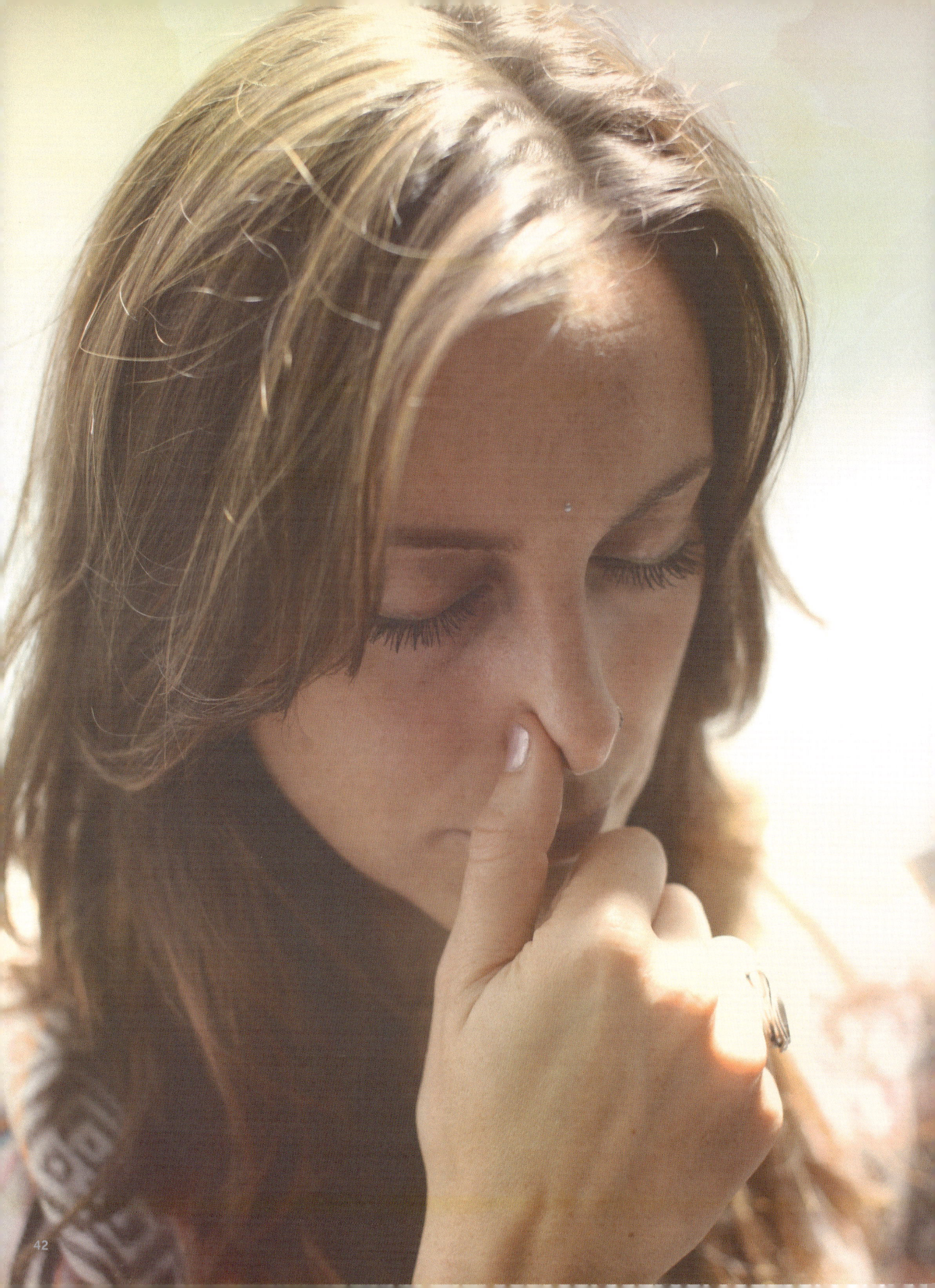

PRANAYAMA

LEFT NOSTRIL BREATHING

POSITION

Sit with a straight spine and pull the chin in to lock the neck (Jalandhar Bandha). Close the eyes and bring them in and up between the brows – to the Third Eye point. Your left hand sits on your left knee in Gyan Mudra (an energy seal bringing forefinger and thumb together).

BREATH

Close off the right nostril with your right thumb and simply breathe long and deep in and out of the left nostril.

DURATION

Continue this pattern of long, deep breathing for 3-31 minutes.

MANTRA

Sat Nam
(Truth is my identity)

TO END

Inhale, exhale completely, hold the breath out and apply Mula Bandha (squeezing anal, sexual and navel muscles), then relax completely.

COMMENTS

You might like to mentally repeat Sat on the inhale and Nam on the exhale – Sat meaning truth and Nam meaning identity or name.

The left nostril and side of the body is associated with feminine, calming attributes and corresponds with the right side of the brain.

Teachers, you can use 3-11 minutes as a pranayama exercise before the kriya.

15 minutes will turn this into a deep meditation.

#embodyyoursoulpurpose
@roisinallanakiernan

KRIYA
FOR THE NEGATIVE MIND

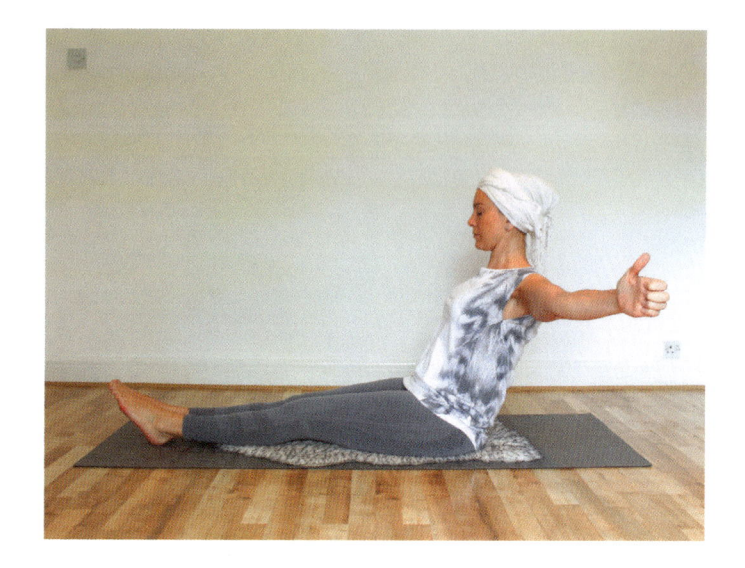

1. So Hung - I Am... 3 Minutes

Instructions: Sit with the legs out in front, arms reaching to the sides, with fingers on the pads, thumbs up. Lean back as far as you can, keeping the back straight – feel your navel engage. Eyes are nine tenths closed. In this position, inhale four equal parts, mentally chanting 'So So So So' then exhale in four equal parts, mentally chanting 'Hung Hung Hung Hung'.

To End: Inhale and close the eyes then exhale and relax the arms. Sit cross-legged, let the breath relax and rest a moment, focussing at the Brow Point.

Benefits: This engages your navel (your will power) to connect with the mantra - So Hung, which simply means, I Am. It also regulates the breath and, therefore, the respiratory system.

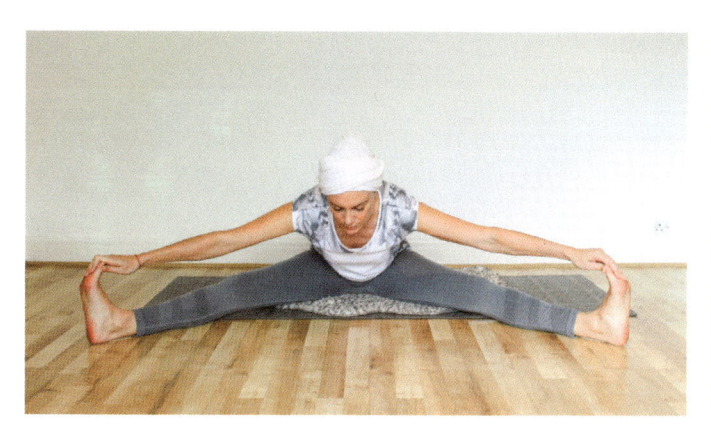

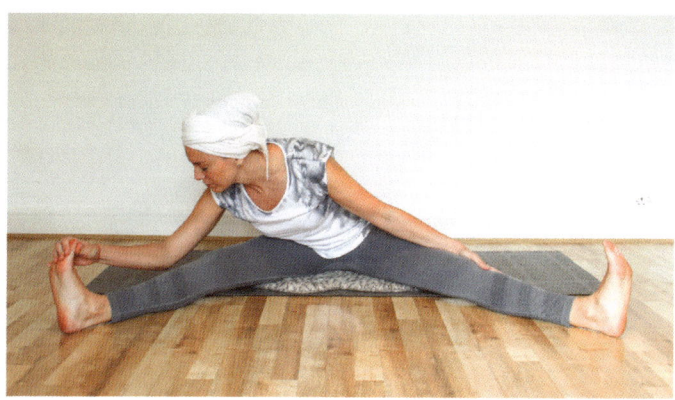

2. Moving Wide Leg Stretch 2 Minutes

Instructions: Stretch your legs out wide in front and take hold of your toes or as far along the legs as you can. Then, keeping hold of your toes, inhale chest up in the centre then exhale down over your left leg; inhale centre, exhale down centre; and continue alternating with inhales and exhales in the centre between each leg. End down in the centre.

Benefits: This strengthens and stretches the spine and muscles of the back. It also works on the hamstrings and inner thighs, opens the hips, the torso and ribcage and increases lung capacity and circulation, whilst invigorating the nervous system.

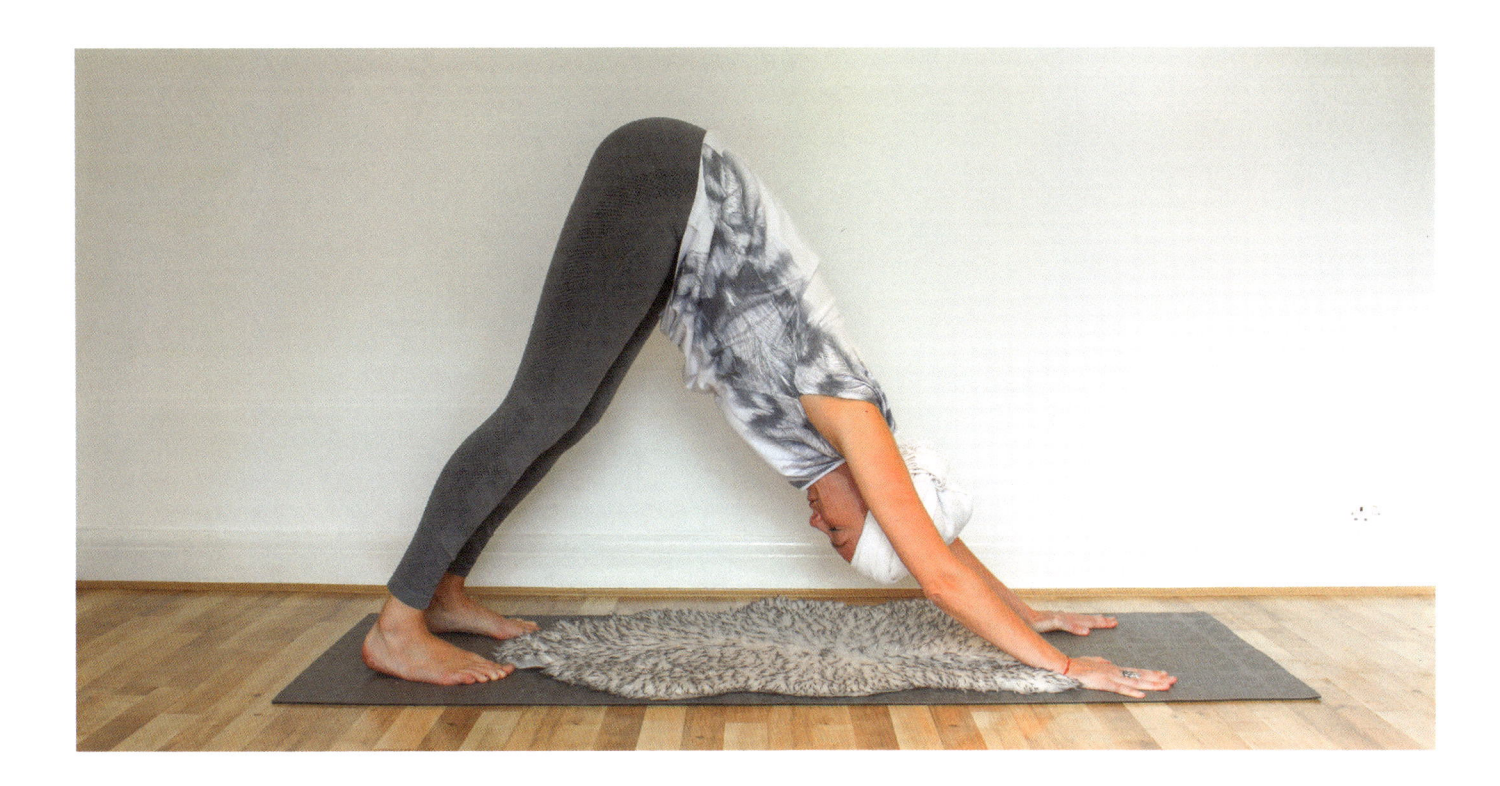

3. Triangle Pose - (Down Dog) 3 Minutes

Instructions: Come onto your hands and knees – wrists under shoulders and knees under hips. Spread your fingers and tuck your toes under, then push up into a triangle-like shape. Push back with your hands, let the chest drop down and hips rise up. You might like to bend the knees at first, bending one after the other to deepen the hamstring stretch. Breathe long and deep.

To End: This works on the sciatic (life) nerve, the sex nerve in the inner thighs, your lower back, the nervous system, shoulders and navel point. You might find yourself shaking in this position – that's the nervous system under pressure, which we want to do in order to strengthen it.

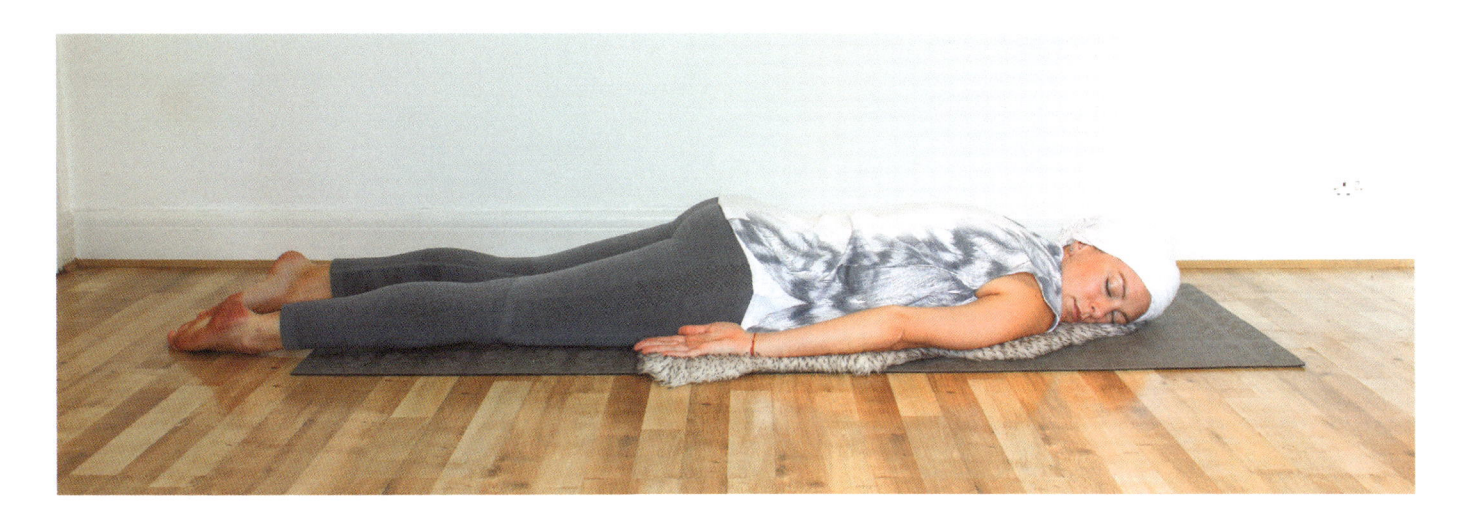

4. Body Survey Rest 1 Minute

Instructions: Come down onto your hands and knees after the last pose, then ease onto your stomach. Turn your head to the side, let your arms rest by your sides and take a moment to survey the body for tension. Feel where you're holding on (where there's tension) and choose to relax.

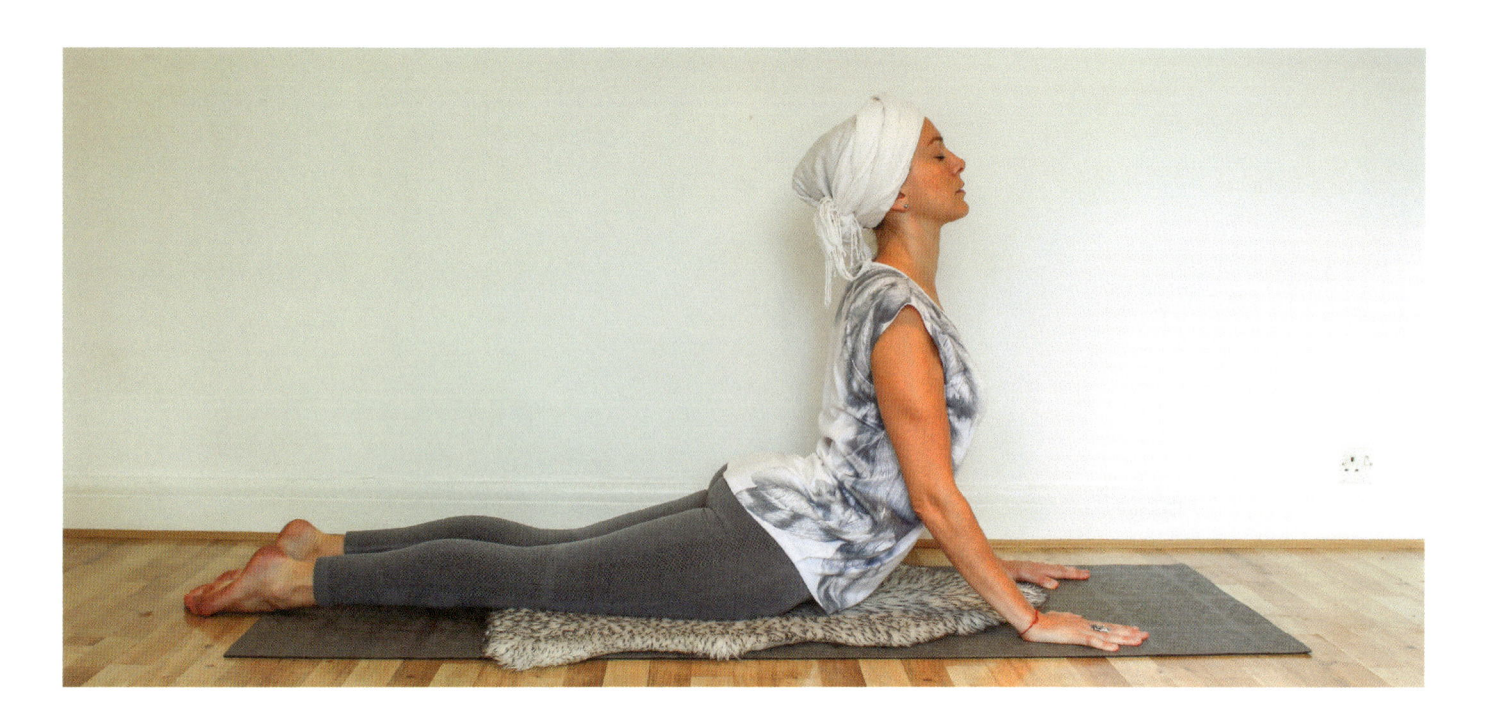

5. Cobra 3 Minutes

Instructions: On your stomach, bring your hands under shoulders, engage your abdomen muscles and lower back, lifting your upper body, before pushing back with the hands. Lift your chest, roll the shoulders back and gently allow the neck to follow the curve of the spine. An alternative option is to rest on the elbows (directly under shoulders) with the hands straight out.

To End: stay in the position and inhale then exhale, hold the breath out and apply Mula Bandha (squeeze anal, sexual and navel). Then release the lock, inhale and slowly lower yourself on the exhale.

Benefits: Strengthens the spine; stretches open the chest and lungs, shoulders and abdomen; firms the buttocks; and can soothe sciatica.

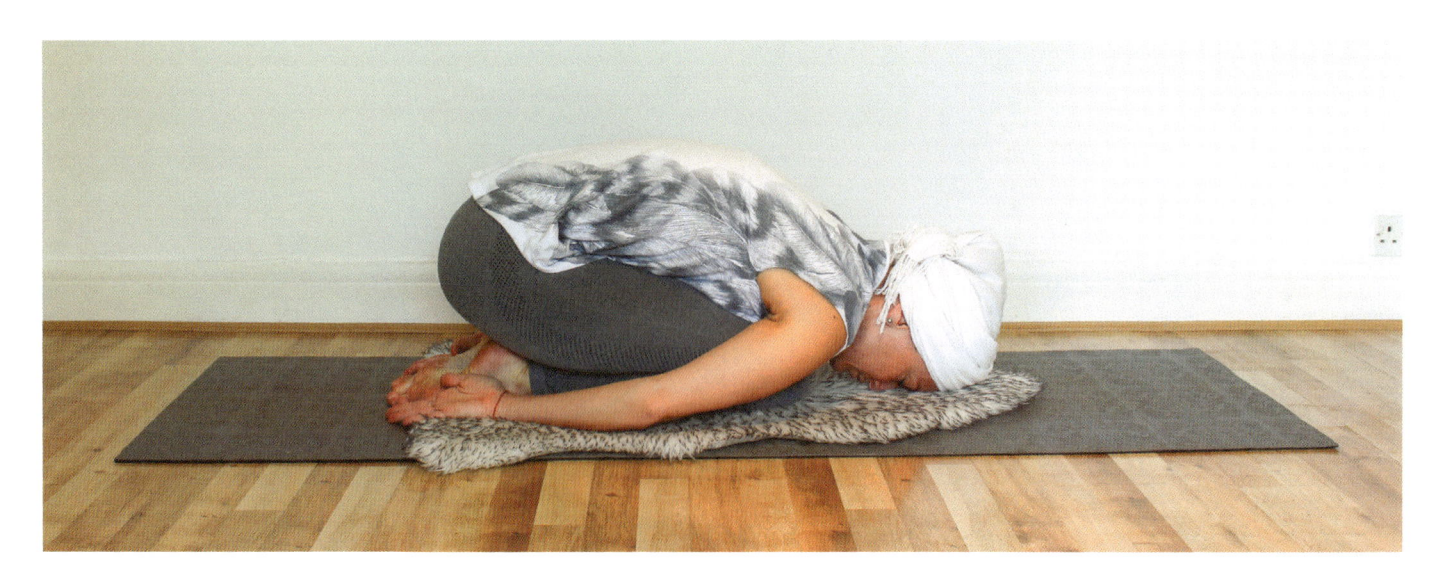

6. Baby Pose 1 Minute

Instructions: Sit back into your heels, knees bent and toes kept down. Rest your forehead on the mat and rest your arms by your sides. Relax.

Benefits: This calms the mind, elongates the lower back, opens the hips and is good for digestion.

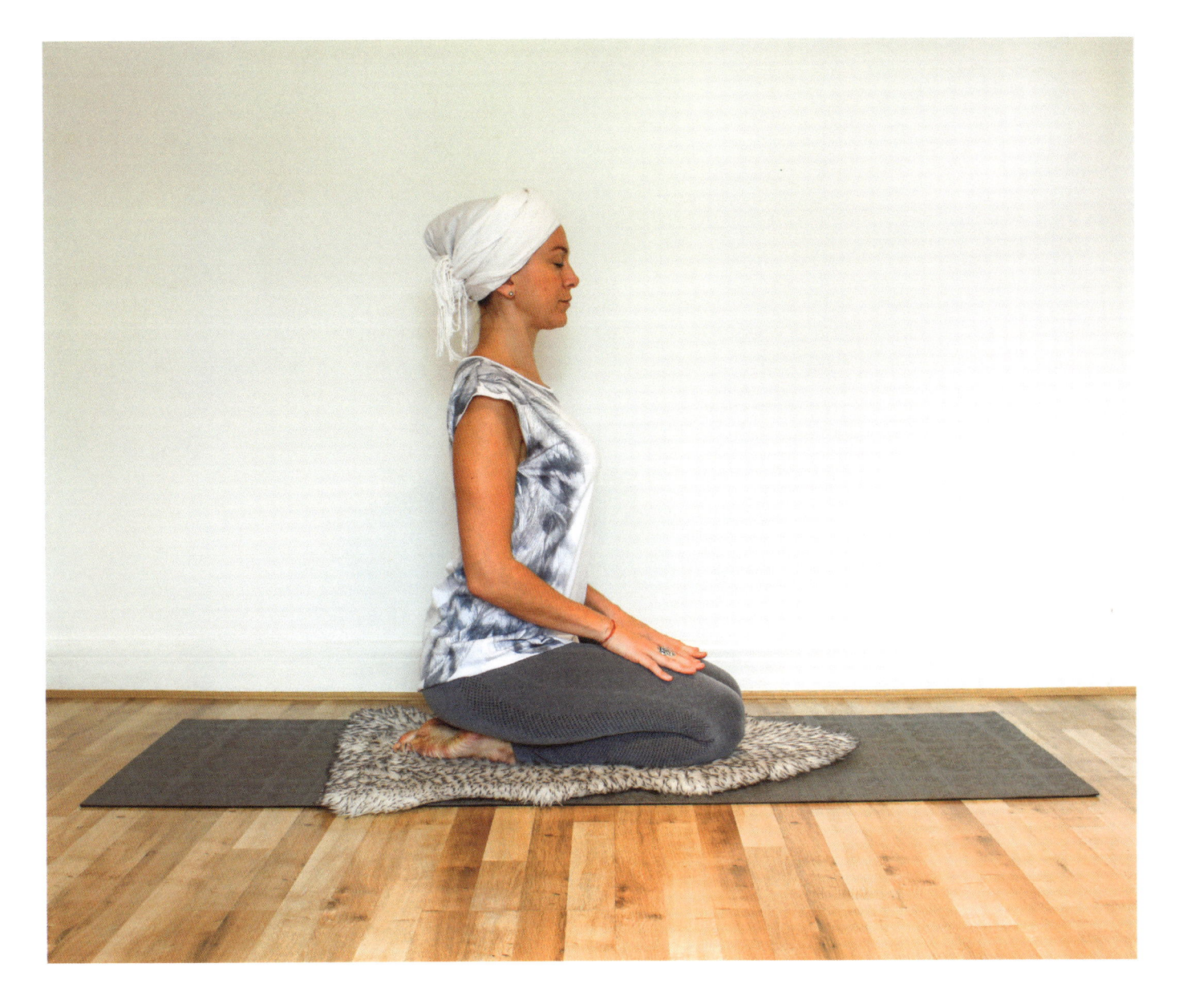

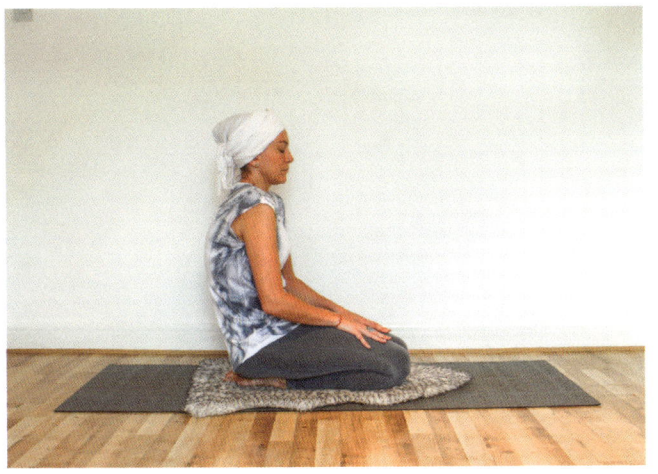

7. Spinal Flex with Held Breath 3 Minutes

Instructions: Sit on your heels, if possible (otherwise, just make sure your spine can be straight and you have room to move). Place your tongue on the gum line of the top teeth and press gently. Then, taking a big inhale, holding and keeping the head in line with the base of the spine, flex your torso forwards and backwards for as long as you're able. Then, return to a central spinal position, exhale and begin again.

Benefits: This strengthens the lungs, increases aerobic ability and rejuvenates the system.

MEDITATION
FOR THE NEGATIVE MIND

POSITION

Sit with a straight spine and bring your hands into a 'cup' at the heart centre – right hand resting in the palm of the left. Your fingers will cross over each other. Elbows relax at the sides. Keep your eyes slightly open and look down into your 'cup'.

BREATH

Inhale long and deep through the nose then exhale through rounded lips into your hands.

DURATION

11 - 31 minutes

TO END

Exhale completely and hold the breath out as you lock in the navel point. Bring your awareness to each vertebra of the spine until you can feel it stiff as a rod. Then inhale powerfully, exhale completely, and repeat 3-5 times before relaxing completely.

COMMENTS

As you inhale, bring to mind any negative or distracting thoughts and then exhale them out. This clears the subconscious of unwanted, negative or fearful thoughts. Once the protective nature of the Negative Mind is balanced, then it's capable of discerning when real protection is necessary. This is a meditation and posture of calm and humility.

#embodyyoursoulpurpose
@roisinallanakiernan

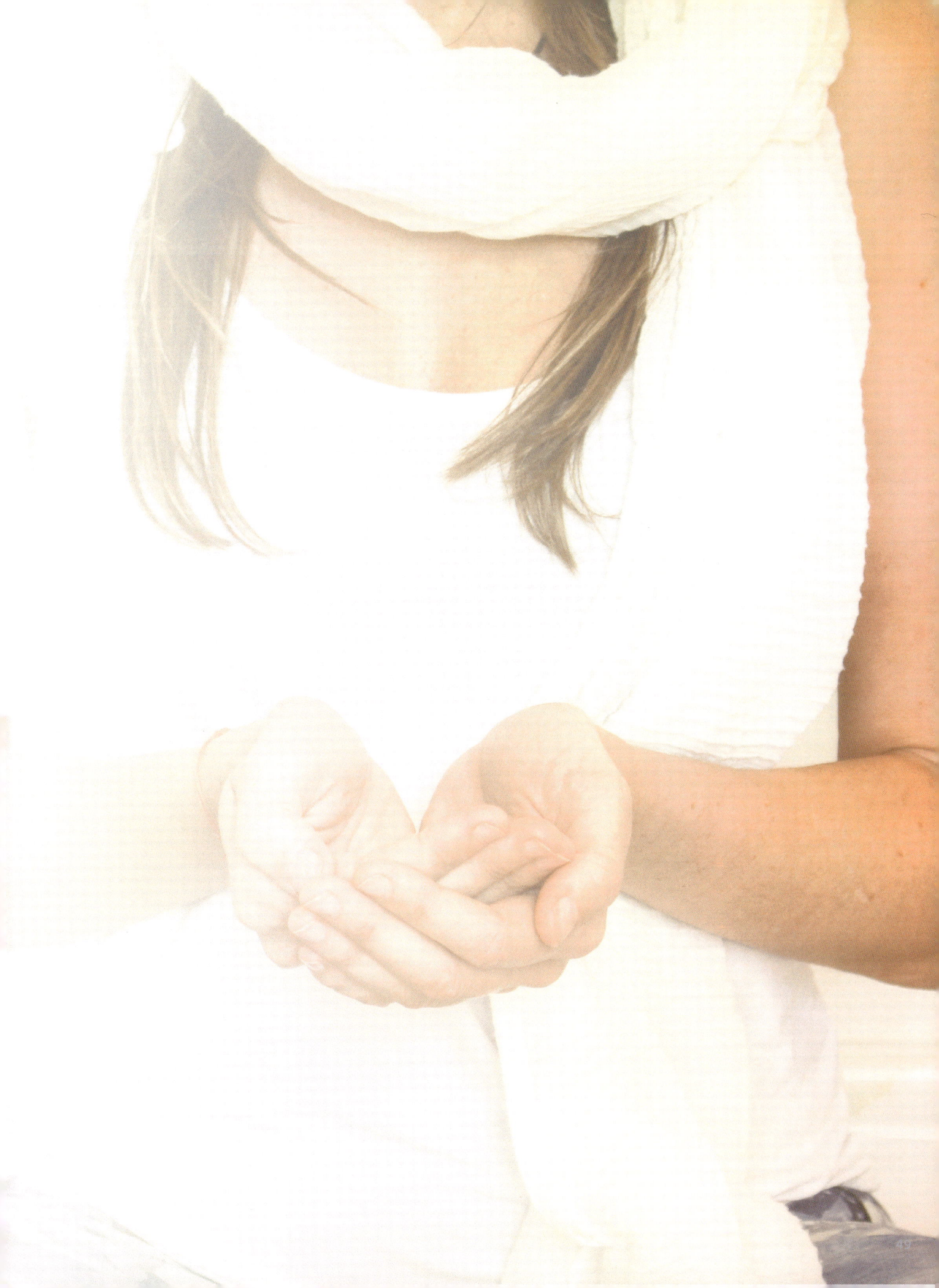

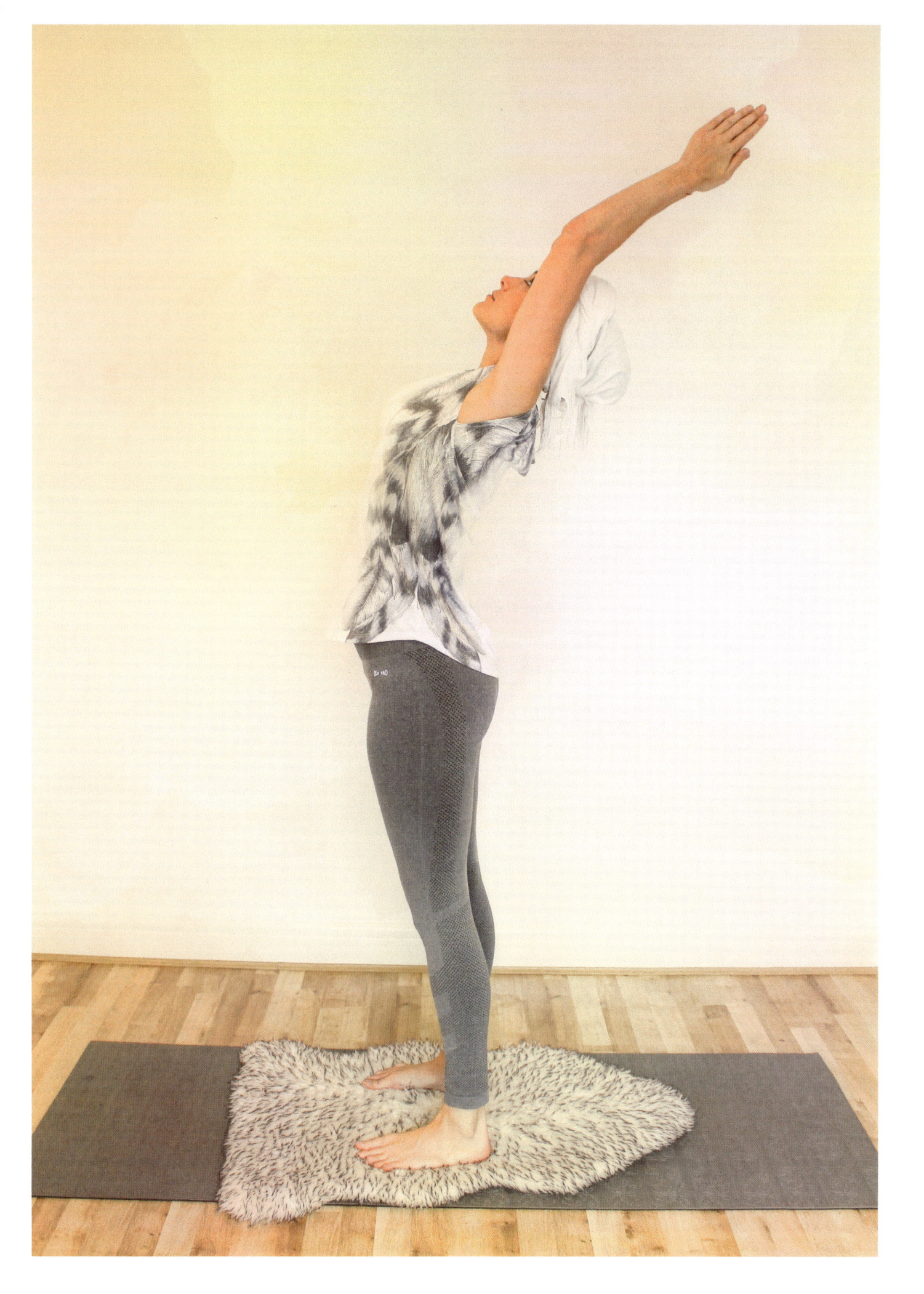

3

THE PROJECTIVE (POSITIVE) MIND

BALANCE INDIVIDUAL WILL WITH DIVINE WILL

A positive mental attitude helps us to achieve but then we must learn to trust and let go, with good humour, secure in the knowledge that all will work out as it should.

#embodyyoursoulpurpose
@roisinallanakiernan

THE PROJECTIVE (POSITIVE) MIND
BALANCE INDIVIDUAL WILL WITH DIVINE WILL

You are powerful – you have the ability, through the Projective Mind, to manifest your life as you wish. But, you have to remember to balance your individual will with divine will. Your inner fire or will gets manifestation in motion but then you have to trust and let go, with good humour, secure in the knowledge that all will work out as it should.

The first few bodies are very much related to the chakras (energy centres within the body). The first is about security, the second about reproduction and the third about will power. With their corresponding elements being (in order) earth, water and fire.

Consider the law of cause and effect. The Projective Mind is designed to create – individual will can be powerful – but there will always be an effect. Too much fire and you or another might get burnt. On the flip side, not enough fire can create a feeling of hopelessness - you might feel as if you've no say over your life, or you might foolishly rush into matters without considering the risks.

When balanced, the Projective Mind brings about good humour. You've carefully put in your work (individual will) but know that divine will is also at play, so you're in trust and ready for what will be. In this way, there's an effortless hope that follows, even when situations don't work out the way you'd planned. This is because you know that everything is happening for you as it should and that you have the strength to work through it.

Equality is the ultimate virtue of the Projective Mind. The number three takes you out of the duality of two and offers an opportunity for structure. But again, balance is key. Control can easily become an issue at the third body – either in terms of being controlling or being controlled, depending, of course, on how much fire is in your belly and how well the projection that pours forth is managed. Choosing to project yourself as a form of self-expression is expansive, but many get caught in the expression-for-others power game, abusing their will to manipulate and gain control.

These power games, your learnt manipulations, create habits within the mind and body – reactions that act like armour, created with protection in mind but actually working to immobilise your growth. Are you the type of person that talks too much or too little? Your individual will, whether weak or strong, can keep you locked in such habits. Habits that boil down to feelings of self-worth. When you're strong in your sense of self, you need not manipulate.

Harnessing individual will through spiritual discipline - working to bring yourself back in line with divine will - can help change unwanted, albeit natural, habits.

When in balance, your three mental bodies will operate together, much like the ultimate equality of three – without comparison or justification – leaving you in trust that all is as it should be.

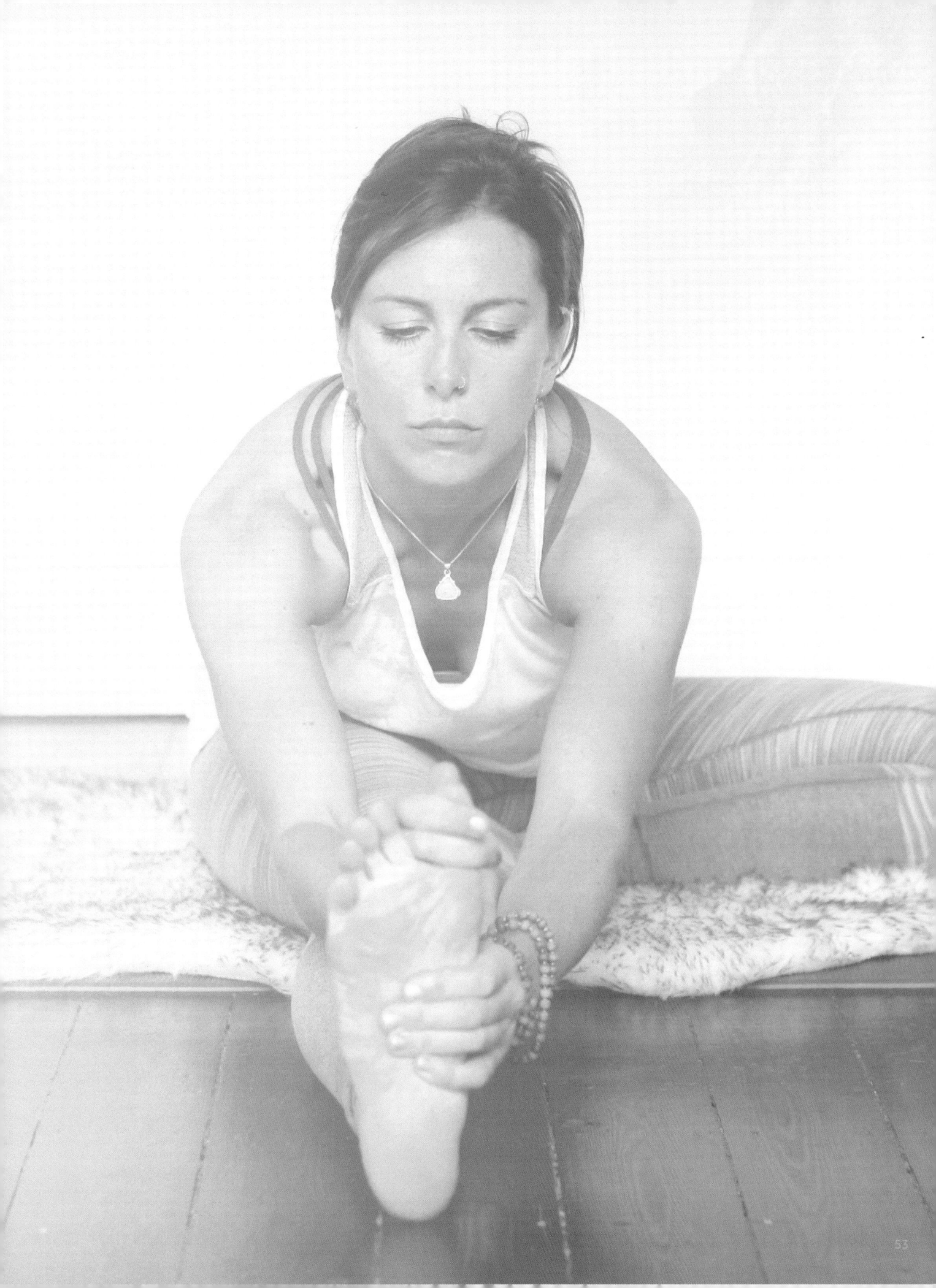

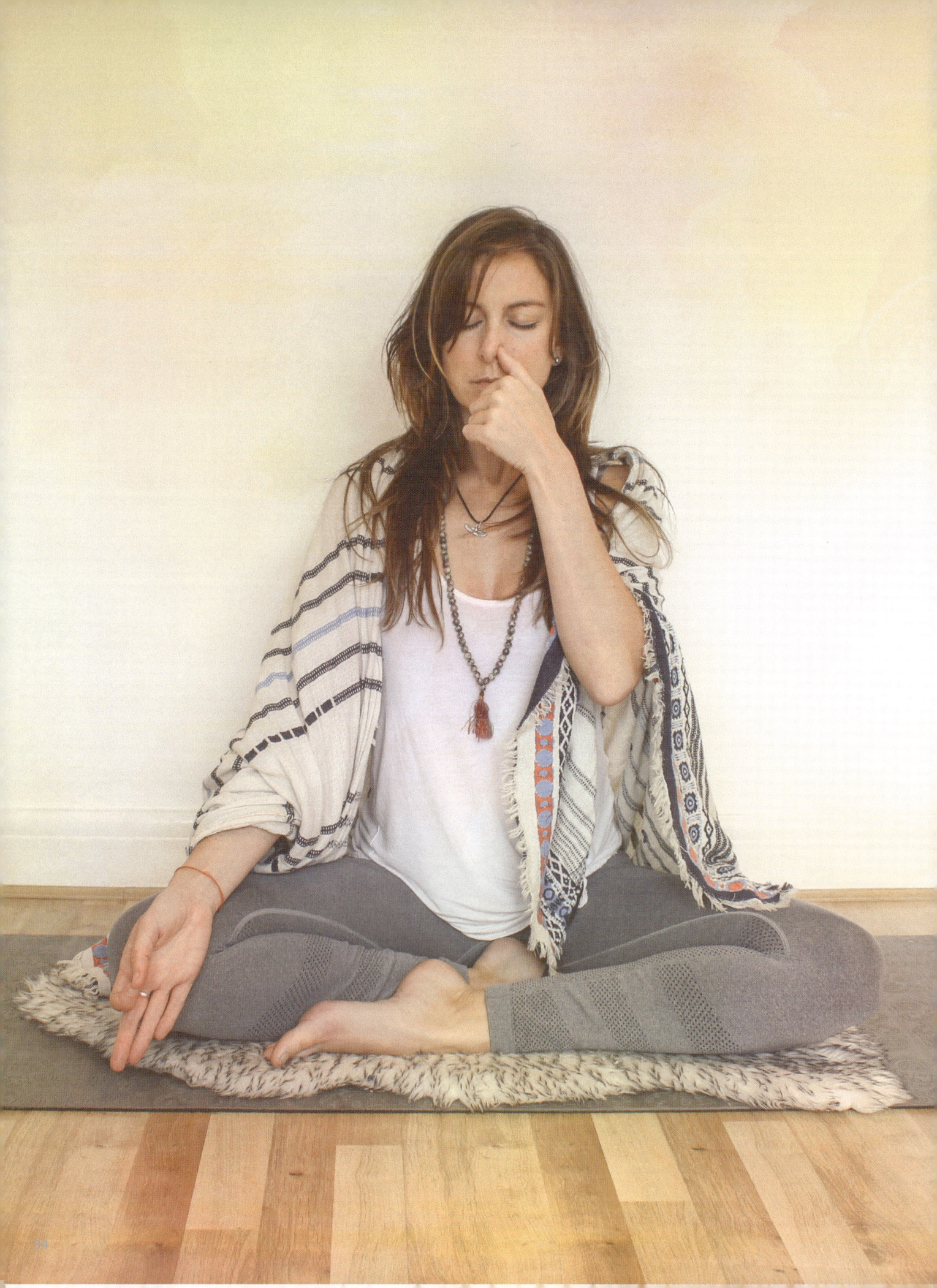

PRANAYAMA
RIGHT NOSTRIL BREATHING

POSITION

Sit with a straight spine and pull the chin in to lock the neck (Jalandhar Bandha). Close the eyes and bring them in and up between the brows – to the Third Eye point. Your right hand rests on your right knee in Gyan Mudra (an energy seal, bringing forefinger and thumb together).

BREATH

Close off the left nostril with your left thumb and simply breathe long and deep in and out of the right nostril.

DURATION

Continue this pattern of long, deep breathing for 3-31 minutes.

TO END

Inhale, exhale completely, hold the breath out and apply Mula Bandha (squeezing anal, sexual and navel muscles), then relax completely.

COMMENTS

You might like to mentally repeat Sat on the inhale and Nam on the exhale – Sat meaning truth and Nam meaning identity or name.

The right side of the body corresponds with the left side of the brain and offers masculine, action-orientated characteristics.

Teachers, you can use 3-11 minutes as a pranayama exercise before the kriya. 15 minutes will turn this into a deep meditation.

#embodyyoursoulpurpose
@roisinallanakiernan

KRIYA
FOR THE POSITIVE MIND

All postures in this Kriya are done for 1-3 minutes each.

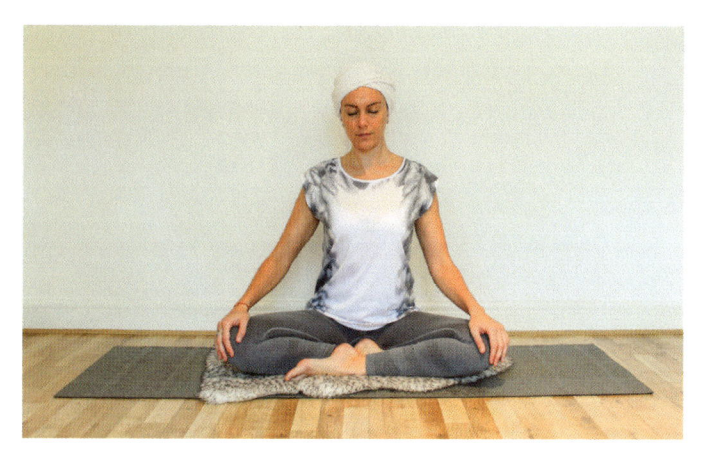

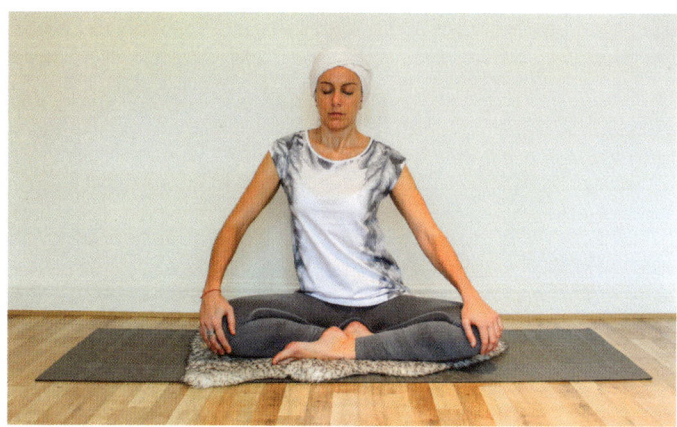

1. Sufi Grinds

Instructions: Sitting with a straight spine, inhale as you start rounding the torso forward, exhaling as you round back. Imagine you're drawing circles around the body with your heart - the head simply follows; relax your neck. The shoulders remain above the hips and the movement is very internal.

Benefits: This warms the spine, easing through any tension and gently massaging the inner organs.

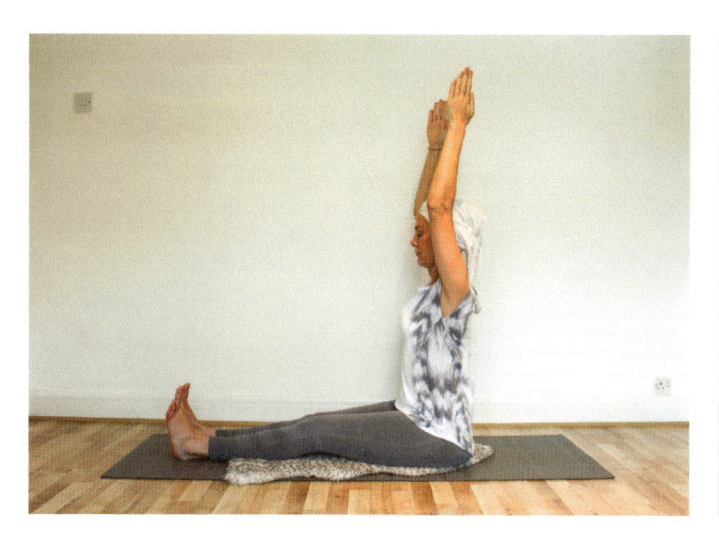

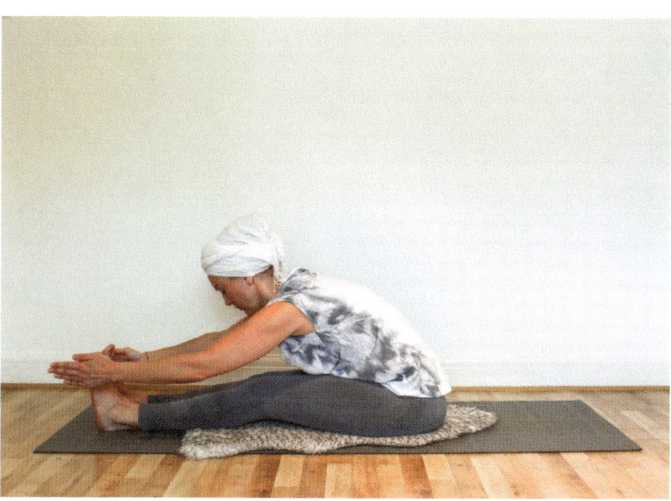

2. Forward Folds

Instructions: Sitting with your feet straight out in front, inhale the arms up (palms facing) and exhale over your feet. Continue; inhaling up, exhaling down.

Benefits: This stretches the sciatic (life) nerve, the hamstrings and lower back. It also gets the spinal fluid flowing.

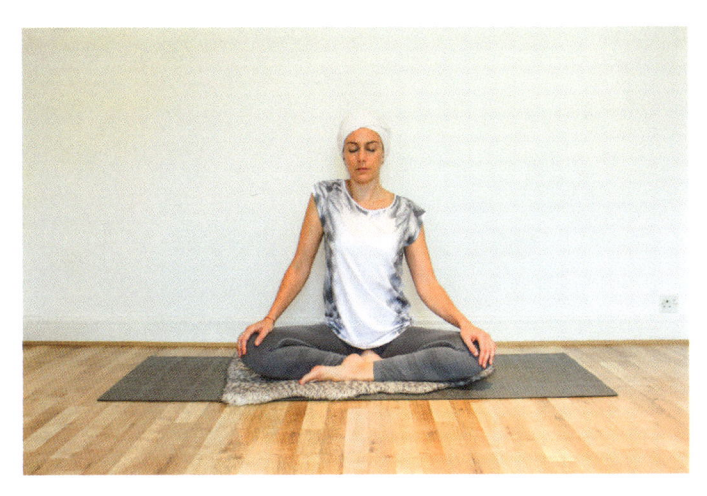

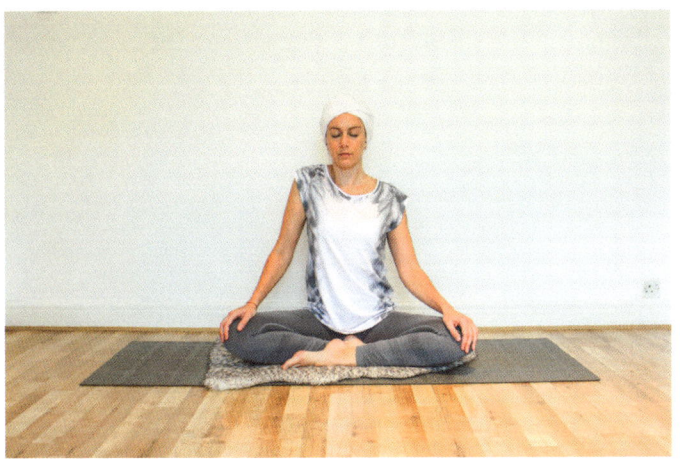

3. Alternate Shoulder Rotations

Instructions: Sitting with your spine straight, inhale the left shoulder forward and up, then exhale back and down before continuing. After one minute, continue with the right shoulder - inhaling forward and up before exhaling back and down. To end, lift both shoulders, hold briefly, and relax.

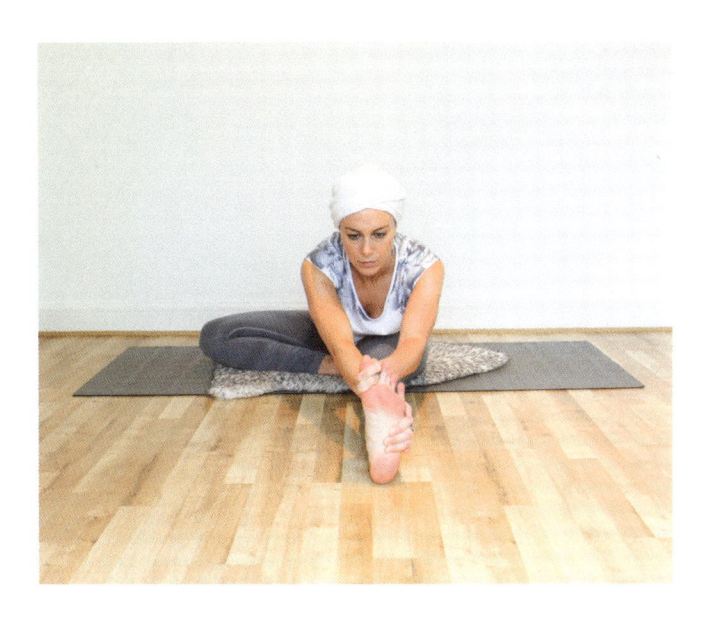

4. Head to Knee Forward Bend with Breath of Fire

Instructions: Start with both legs straight out in front then bring the right foot in towards the groin, resting along the inner left thigh. Then inhale, stretch both arms up and forward fold over the left leg, taking hold of the big left toe if possible. Holding this possible, begin Breath of Fire whilst holding Mula Bandha. Eyes remain open, looking at the big toe.

Benefits: This offers a good stretch for the sciatic (life) nerve and hamstrings. Combined with Breath of Fire, it also rejuvenates the system.

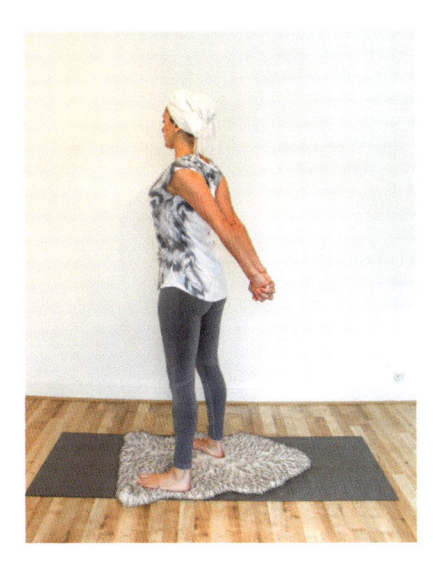

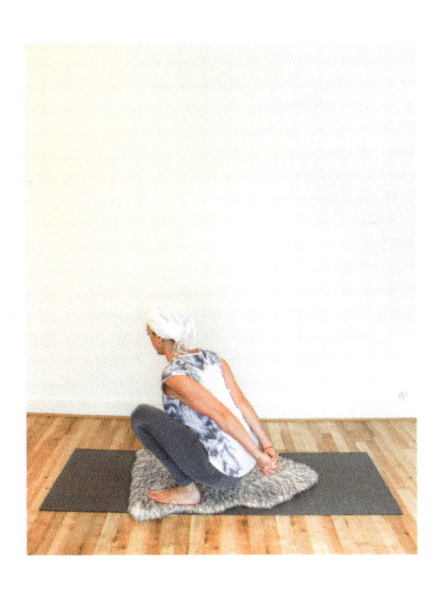

5. Squats

Instructions: Stand and interlace your fingers in Venus Lock behind the back. Inhale as you lift the hands with straight arms. Exhale as you relax the arms and squat down into the thighs.

Benefits: Opens the shoulders and strengths buttocks and thighs.

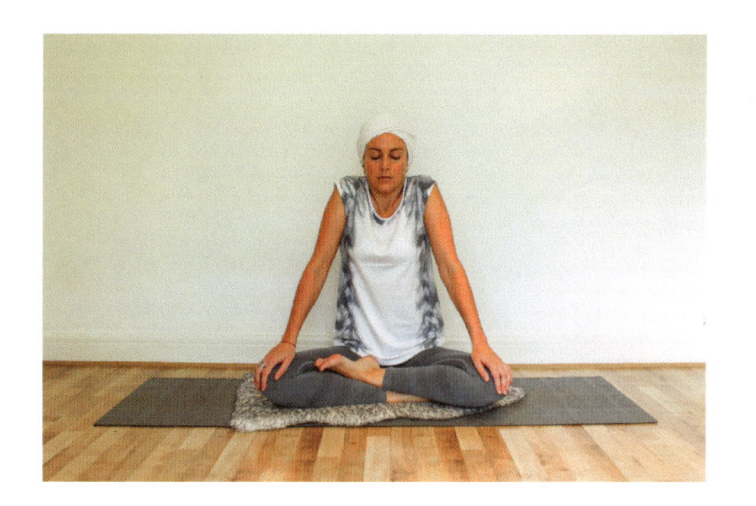

6. Double Shoulder Rotations

Instructions: Sitting with your spine straight, inhale the shoulders forward and up, then exhale back and down before continuing. Then, on the second round, take your shoulders in the opposite direction – inhaling back and up and exhaling forward and down. To end, inhale and raise both shoulders up, hold for a few seconds, exhale, and relax.

7. Legs Up with Breath of Fire

Instructions: Lie on your back and bring both legs up 90degrees, feet together.. Hold and do Breath of Fire.

Benefits: This is relaxing and enlivening at the same time. It stretches your hamstrings and lower back, strengthens your nervous system and rejuvenates the body with the breath.

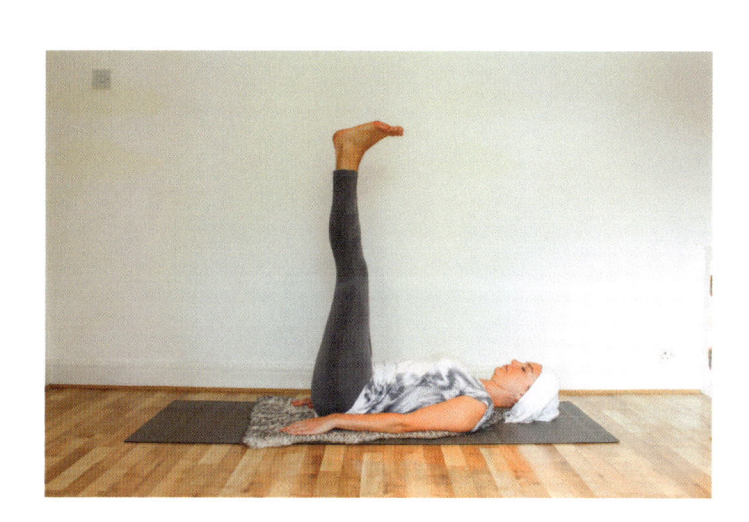

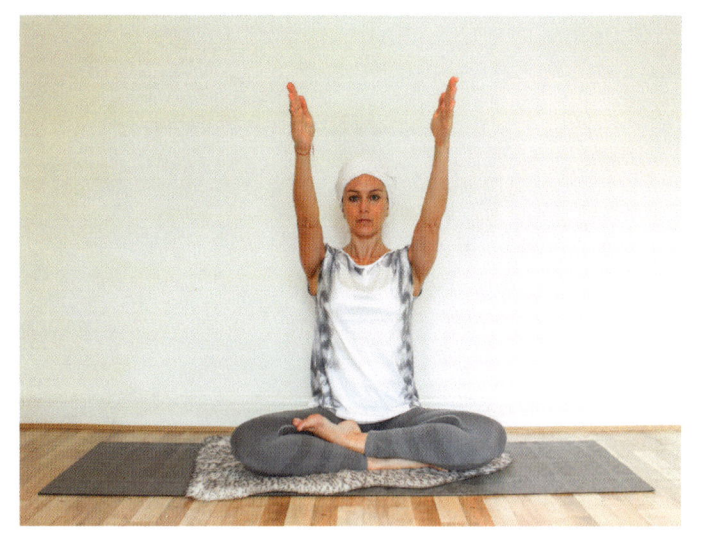

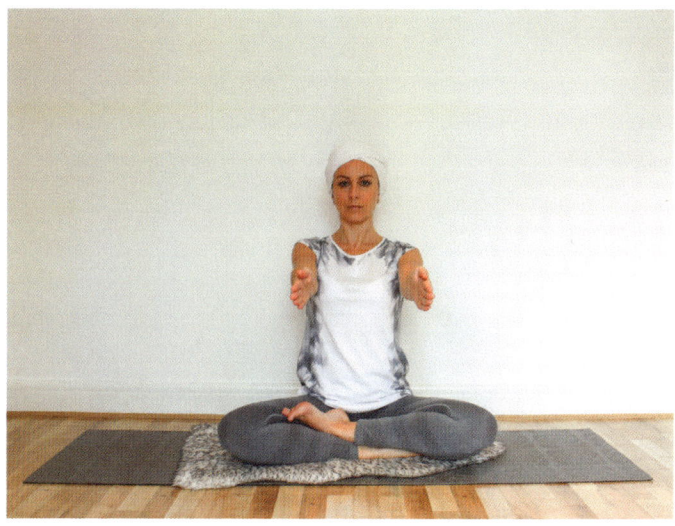

8. Hand Chop

Instructions: Sitting with a straight spine, bring your hands out in front, palms facing. Inhale them up to 60 degrees and then exhale down to 30 degrees. Keep the arms straight and the palms facing each other. Build it up to be a rapid movement.

Benefits: Strengthens the navel and cuts through any stagnant/held/non-positive emotions.

9. Miracle Bend

Instructions: Stand with the feet hip distance apart and raise your arms up into prayer above the head. Look up, contract the navel and lower back, and stretch back. Stay steady and strong at your core – be careful of your back; don't over-do it. Holding this position, begin Breath of Fire.

Benefits: This opens the heart, strengthens the core and clears negativity.

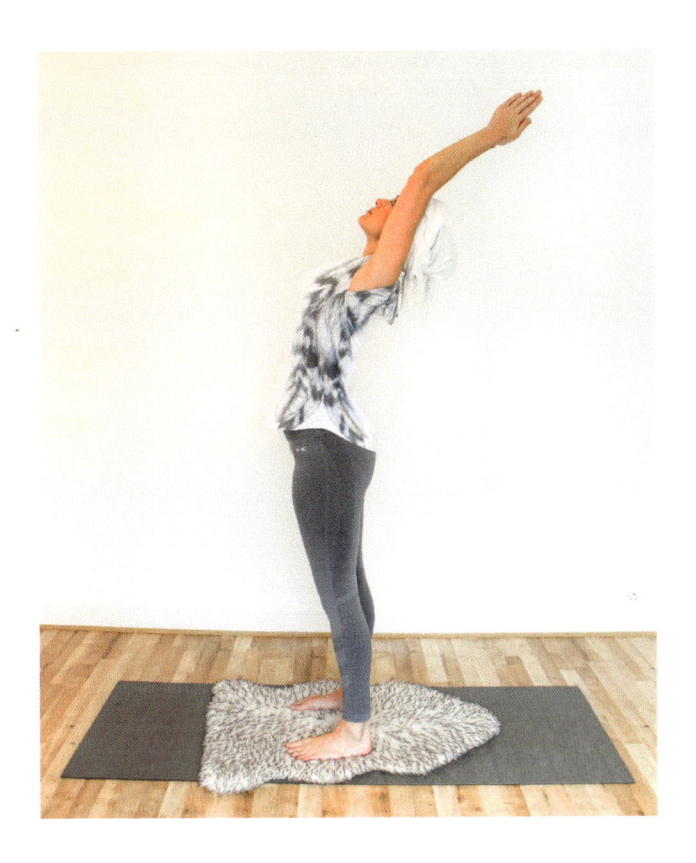

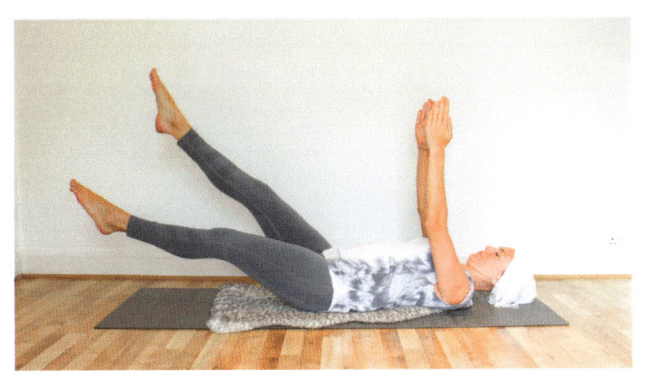

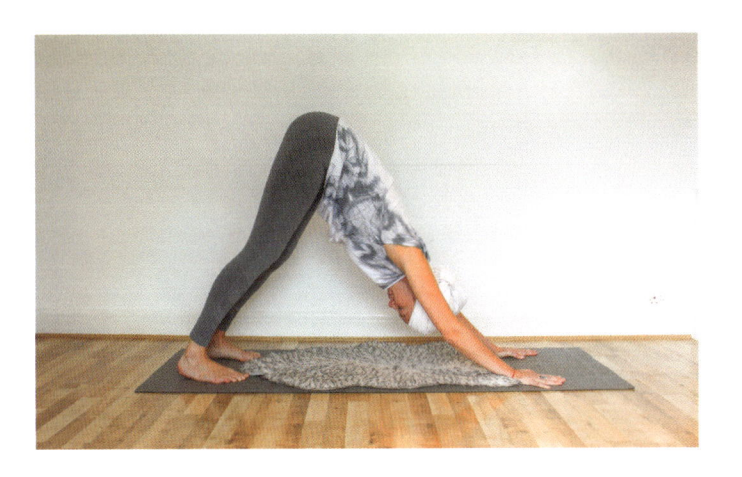

10. Alternate Leg Lifts

Instructions: Lie on your back and bring both legs up to 30 degrees, then alternately lift each leg up 60 degrees. Inhaling one up to 60 and exhaling the other down to 30 – like scissors. Both legs remain off the ground during this exercise. The arms are up perpendicular to the floor with palms facing each other. Alternatively, you can bring your hands, palms facing down, under your buttocks to support your lower back.

Benefits: This strengthens the core, glutes, hips and legs.

11. Triangle Pose (Down Dog)

Instructions: Start on your hands and knees (wrists under shoulders and knees under hips). Spread your fingers wide and tuck your toes under. Then push up, straightening arms and legs, into a triangle position. Push back with the hands, let the chest drop down and hips tilt up. You might wish to bend the legs initially, bending one at a time to get deeper into the stretch on each leg. Let the head drop down – relax your neck. In this position, inhale four sniffs to full and then exhale smoothly in one go. Your eyes should be focussed towards the navel.

Benefits: This works on the sciatic (life) nerve, the sex nerve in the inner thighs, your lower back, the nervous system, shoulders and navel point. You might find yourself shaking in this position – that's the nervous system under pressure, which we want to do in order to strengthen it.

MEDITATION
FOR THE POSITIVE MIND

POSITION

Sitting with a straight spine, curl your ring and little fingers into each palm and bend the thumbs over them. The first and second fingers remain upright. Press the elbows and shoulders back firmly but comfortably.

Close your eyes and roll them in and up to the Third Eye, between the brows.

Mentally then, start to pulse out from your Third Eye the mantra 'Saa, Taa, Naa, Maa' (meaning infinity, life, death, rebirth – the cycle of life).

MANTRA

Saa, Taa, Naa, Maa

BREATH

Breathe long and deep in and out through both nostrils.

DURATION

11 - 62 minutes

TO END

Inhale deeply and exhale three times. Then open and close the fists several times before relaxing.

COMMENTS

This meditation opens the heart centre and the feelings of the positive self. It's said to be a gesture of happiness that has been practised by many great spiritual teachers, including Buddha and Jesus. The hand mudra is a symbol for blessings and prosperity and the mantra works to bring balance to the psyche.

#embodyyoursoulpurpose
@roisinallanakiernan

61

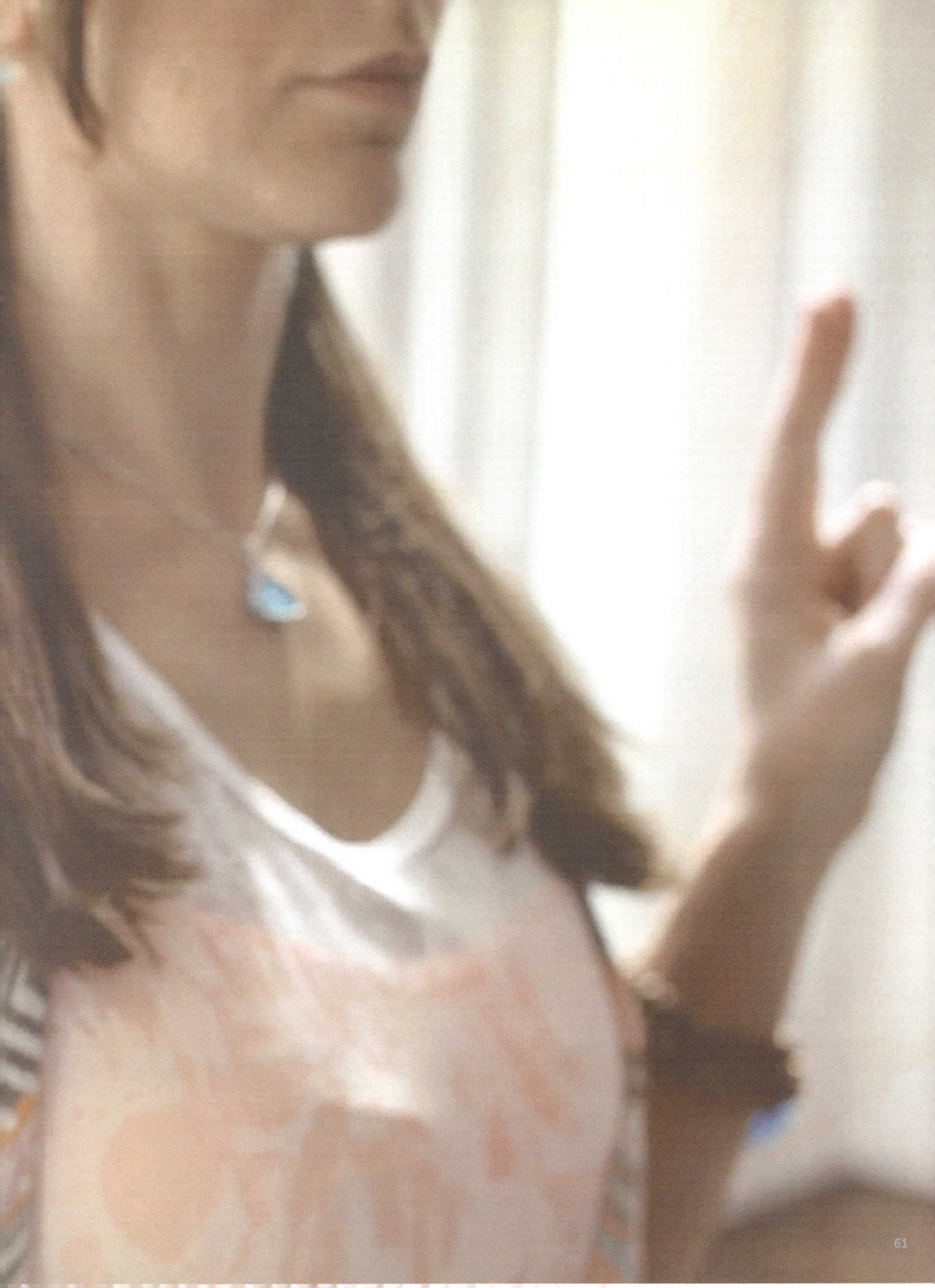

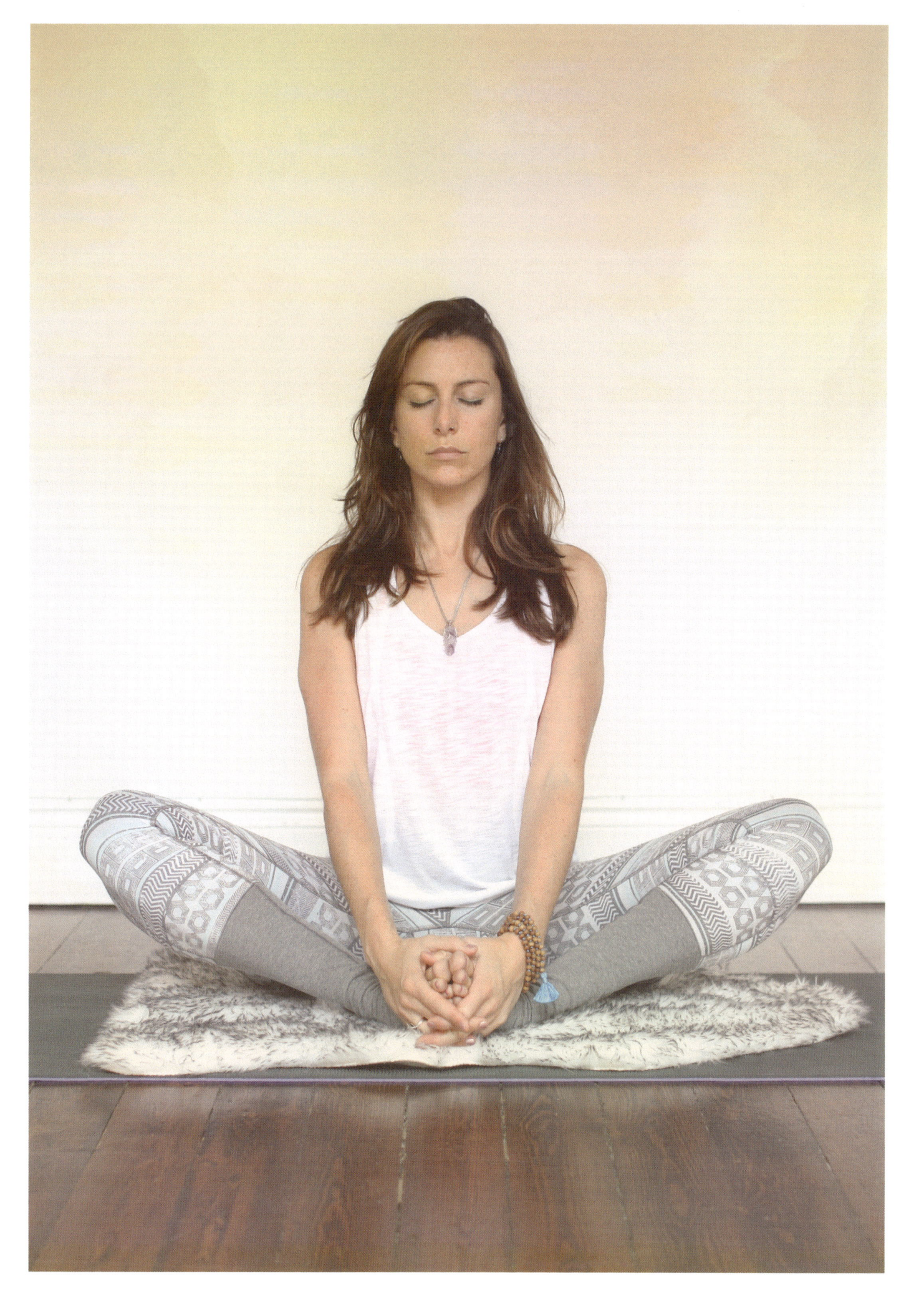

4

THE MEDITATIVE (NEUTRAL) MIND

BREATHE, THEN ACT

A meditative mind will 'tick-tock' between the pros and cons of each situation and find a place of neutrality between them.

#embodyyoursoulpurpose

@roisinallanakiernan

THE MEDITATIVE (NEUTRAL) MIND
BREATHE, THEN ACT

The way you breathe is key to a neutral or meditative mind.

Through mindful breathing you can give yourself the space to act rather than react. You can manage your responses to people or situations by choosing how to be, with compassion and responsibility.

We all have triggers that remind us of painful past experiences. Triggers that we subconsciously choose to remember and subconsciously design responses to in order to try and protect ourselves. Over time, these create habitual neural pathways and reactions that can recreate negative patterns.

Through the breath, you can create the space for awareness; you can start to notice your triggers and responses; you can retrain your mind not to react; you can choose to act from a place of compassion – for yourself and others. This, in turn, creates real strength – the faith and conviction that comes from truly feeling and understanding yourself.

A meditative or neutral mind will 'tick-tock' between the Positive and Negative Minds – looking at the positives and negatives of a situation - and then find a place of neutrality between them. In this way, a neutral mind will bring balance to the areas where you might be overly-projective or overly-protective.

A neutral consciousness is compassionate, open and malleable. The doubt that arises from this fluidity only exists in relation to trust and that has to start with yourself.

One of the great paradoxes of life and one of the hardest lessons is that you can only be free from your feelings once you've fully experienced them. This also teaches that you can never become habitually neutral – it is a constant process – for feelings constantly change and you have to constantly remain conscious, through the breath and mindfulness.

An evolved neutral mind means you can easily pass through the experience of change in fortune, finance or otherwise. Everything simply is and you work with what you have – taking full responsibility for your choices whilst remaining unattached to the outcome. Moment by moment, breath by breath, with full awareness and compassion.

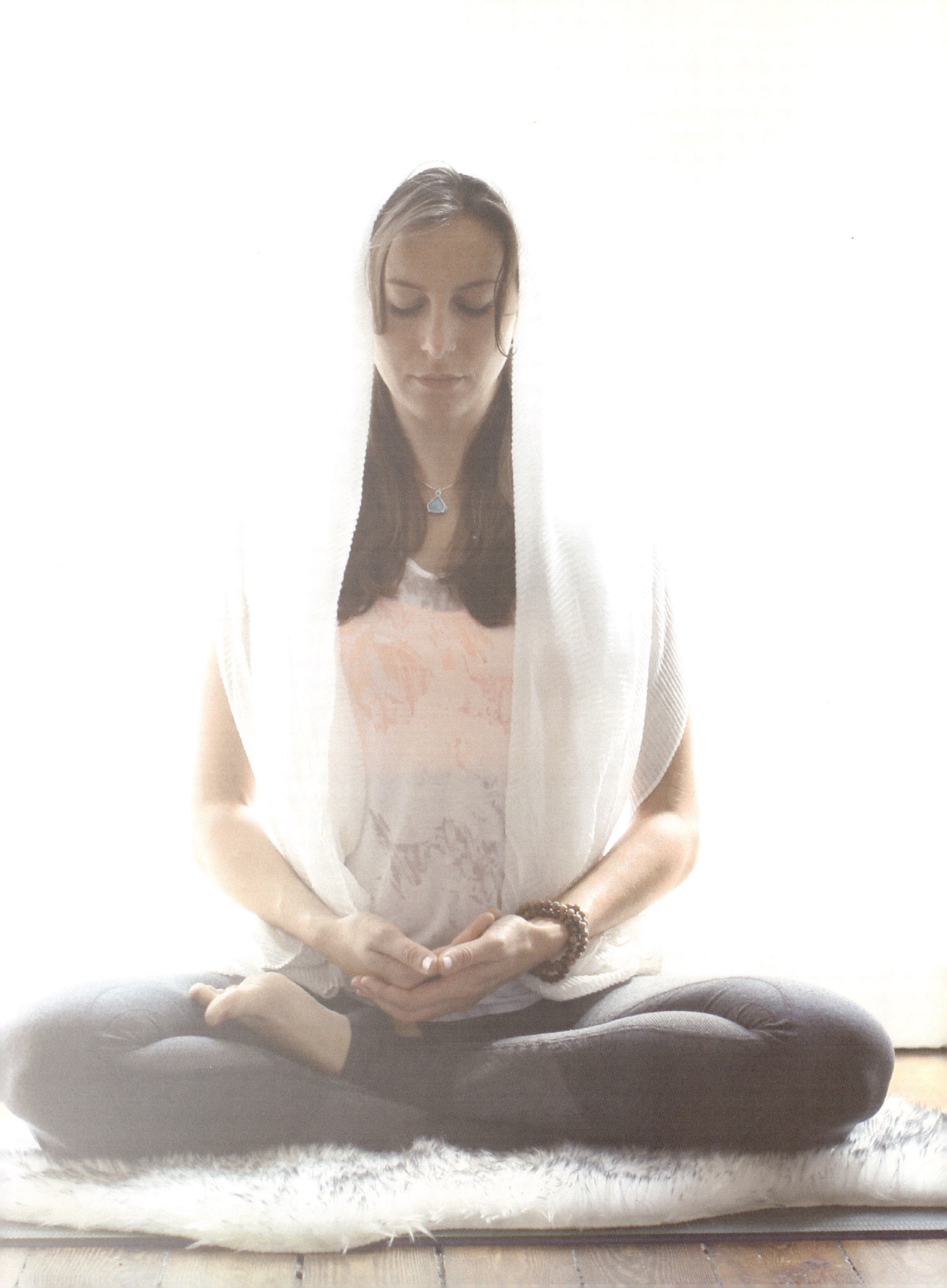

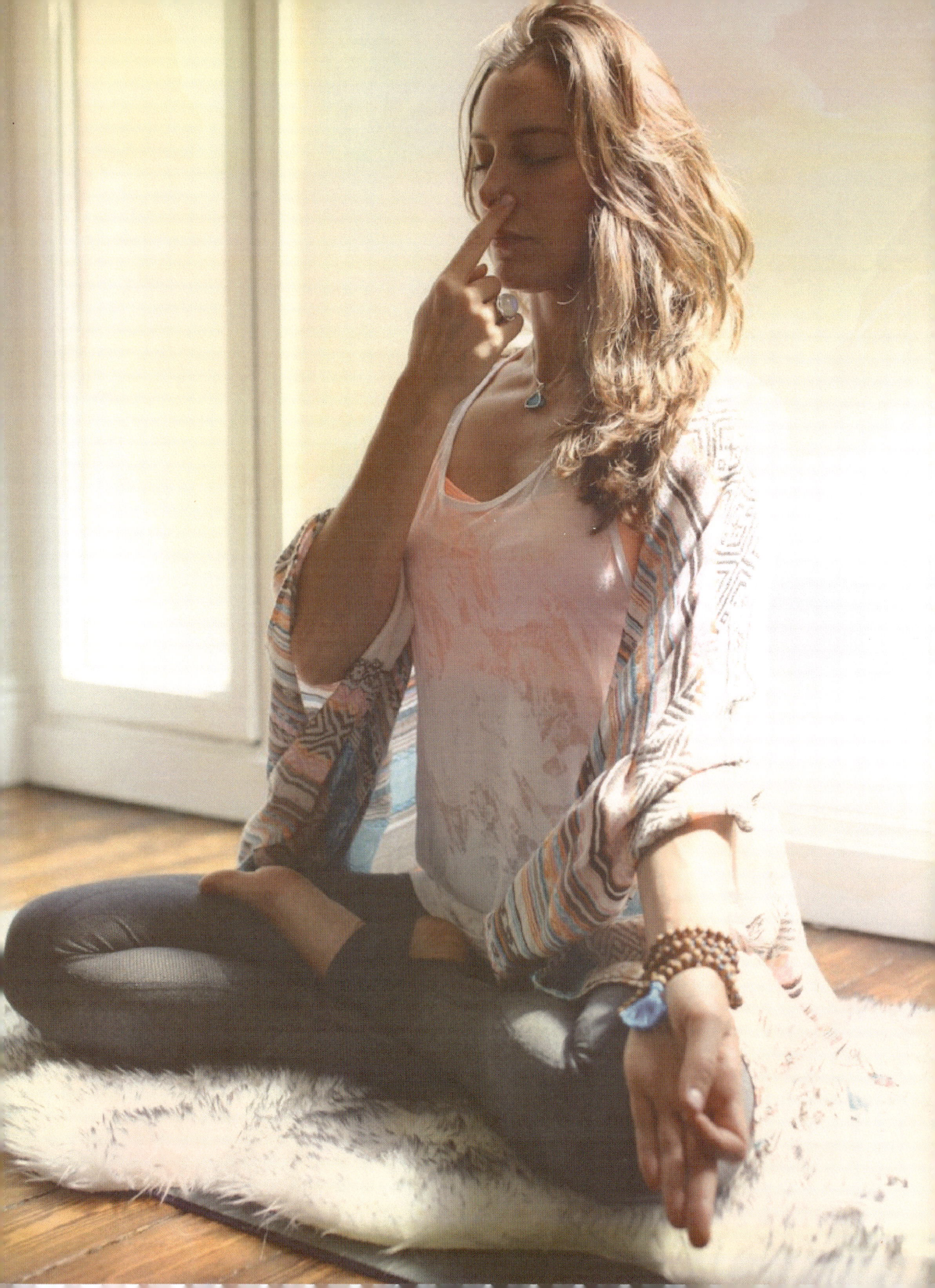

PRANAYAMA

ALTERNATE NOSTRIL BREATHING FOR PERSPECTIVE AND EMOTIONAL BALANCE

POSITION

Sit with a straight spine and pull the chin in to lock the neck (Jalandhar Bandha). Close the eyes and bring them in and up between the brows — to the Third Eye point. Your left hand rests on your knee in Gyan Mudra (an energy seal, bringing forefinger and thumb together).

BREATH

Close off the right nostril with the right thumb. Inhale deeply through the left nostril. When the breath is full hold it for as long as you comfortably can, then close off the left nostril with the index finger, and exhale smoothly through the right nostril. Continue in the opposite direction (inhaling right, holding and exhaling left) and repeat continuously. The breaths are complete, continuous, and smooth.

DURATION

Continue this pattern of long, deep breathing for 3-31 minutes.

TO END

After an exhale, inhale with both nostrils, exhale completely, hold the breath out and apply Mula Bandha (squeezing anal, sexual and navel muscles). Then relax completely.

COMMENTS

You might like to mentally repeat Sat on the inhale and Naam on the exhale — Sat meaning truth and Naam identity or name.

This is a very balancing breath; bringing emotional, mental and feminine/masculine balance. The left nostril and side of the body is associated with feminine, calming attributes and corresponds with the right side of the brain. The right side and left brain offers masculine, action-orientated characteristics. Alternate nostril breath balances both sides.

Teachers, you can use 3-10 minutes as a pranayama exercise before the kriya. 15 minutes will turn this into a deep meditation.

Practising this pranayama as a meditation for 31 minutes will detoxify and restore the body's nervous system. This is a great practise after intense times of stress or shock.

#embodyyoursoulpurpose
@roisinallanakiernan

KRIYA
FOR THE FOURTH BODY (NEUTRAL MIND)

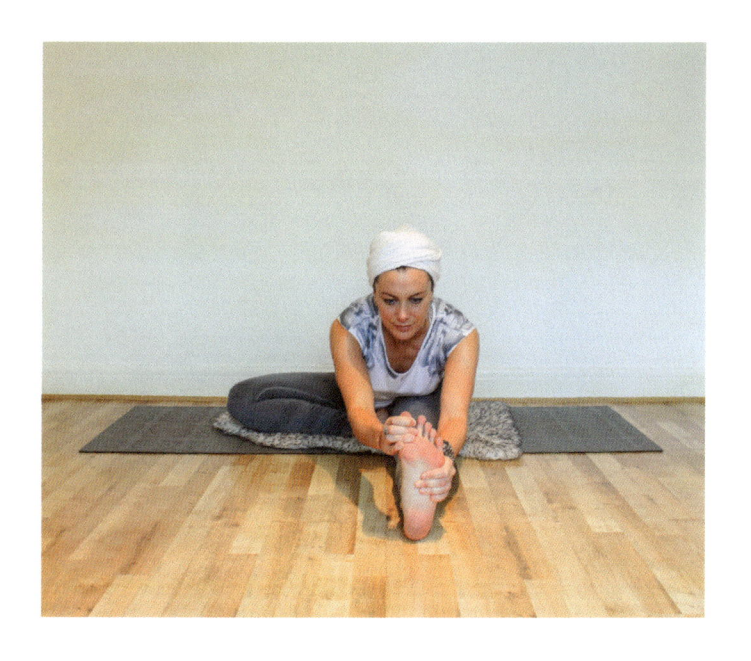

1. Head to Knee Forward Bends

3 Minutes Over Each Leg

Instructions: Start with both legs straight out in front then bring the right foot in towards the groin, resting along the inner left thigh. Inhale, stretch both arms up and forward fold over the left leg, taking hold of the big left toe if possible. Relaxing into this position, begin long, deep breathing. Do both sides.

Benefits: This offers a good stretch for the sciatic (life) nerve and hamstrings. Combined with long, deep breathing, it also revitalises the system.

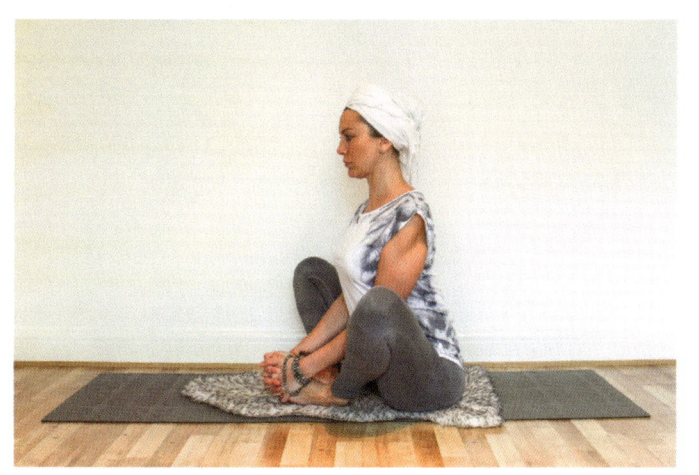

2. Butterfly Pose with Breath of Fire

1 Minute

Instructions: Bring the soles of the feet together in front of you - taking hold of them with the hands and drawing them in as close to you as possible. Then lean forward, keep the head up, and begin a light and fast Breath of Fire (rapidly inhaling and exhaling through the nostrils using your navel as a pump for the breath). To end, inhale, exhale, hold the breath out and apply Mula Bandha. Release it, inhale, and exhale.

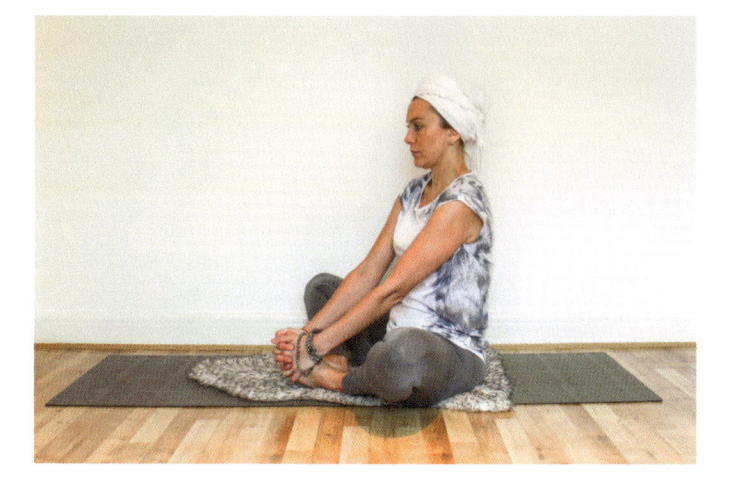

Benefits: This opens the hips, stretches the inner thigh and life nerves (sex and sciatic nerves) and, with Breath of Fire, rejuvenates the system.

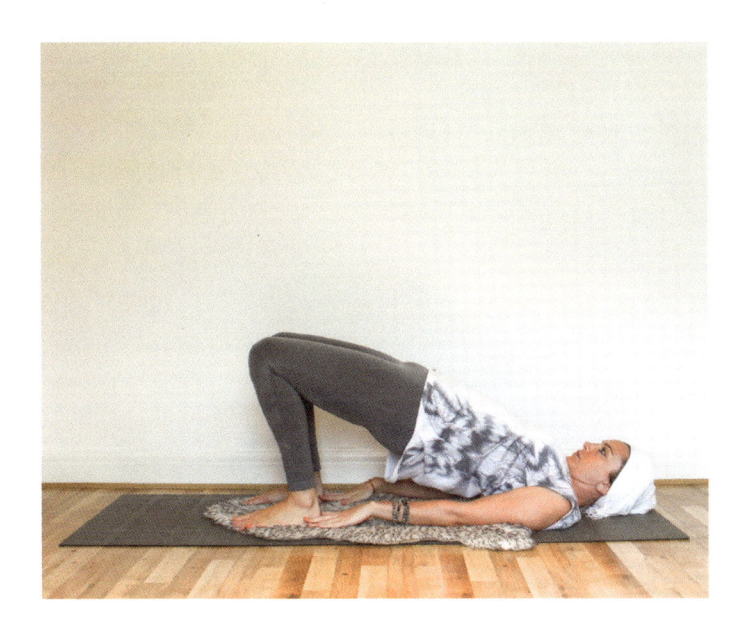

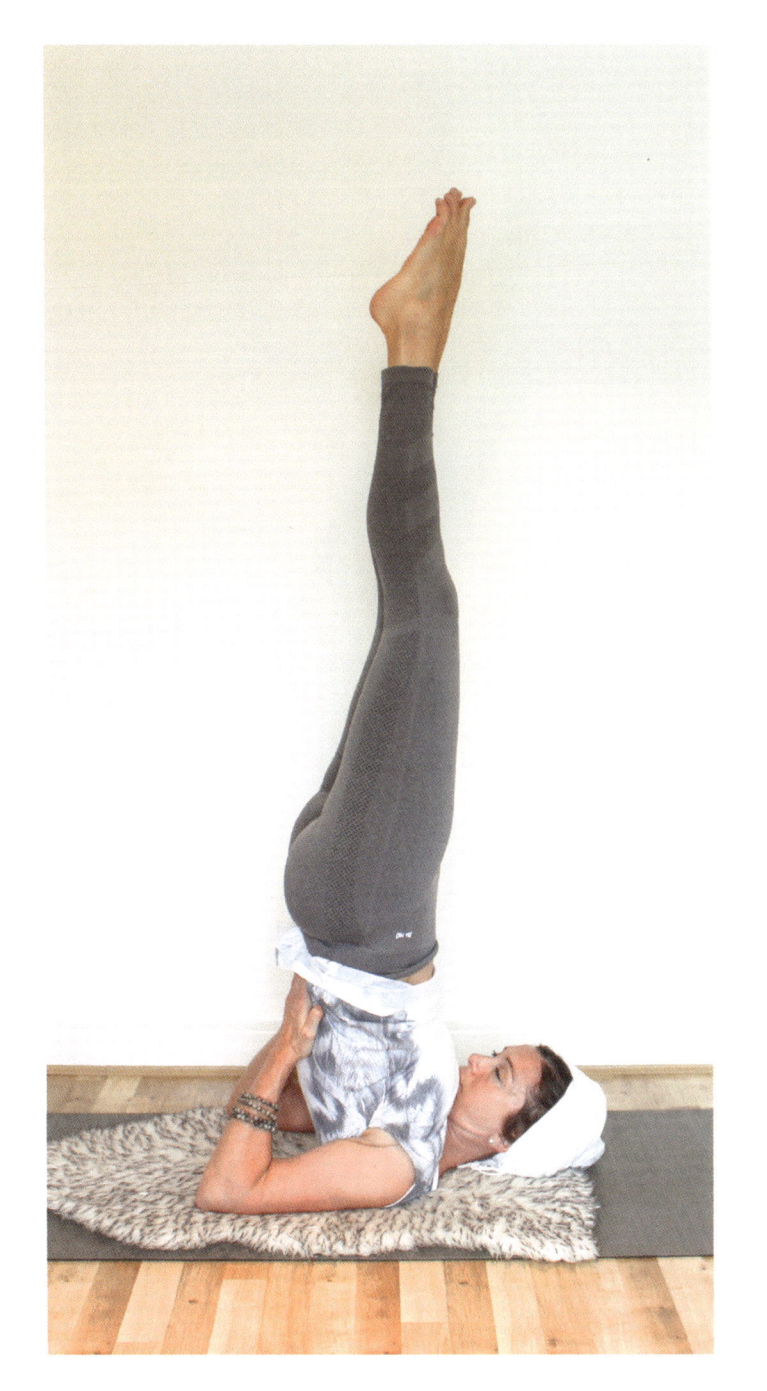

3. Pelvic Lifts 2 Minutes

Instructions: Start by lying down on your back, then bend the knees and bring the feet flat. Reach down and catch the ankles or touch the fingertips against the heels – do what you can. Now, start inhaling as you raise the pelvis high and exhaling as you lower it down. The eyes are closed, focused at the Third Eye (in and up between the brows), but your attention is at the navel.

Benefits: This opens the hips and pelvic bowl and strengthens the lower back, buttocks and pelvic floor muscles.

4. Shoulder Stand 1 Minute

Instructions: Lying on your back, draw the knees up towards your chest, then raise the feet up towards the ceiling. Lift the buttocks as you rise up, drawing the hands under the lower back to support you. Keep the weight in the shoulders – be careful of your neck – and slowly straighten the legs up, pointing the toes towards the ceiling. Hold and concentrate at the Third Eye with long, deep breathing.

To end, ease the feet back over the head into Plow Pose (if able) and then slowly lower yourself, vertebrae by vertebrae down onto your back

Benefits: This is an all-round health tonic – balancing the hormones, strengthening the heart and respiratory systems, soothing the nervous system and increasing strength and flexibility.

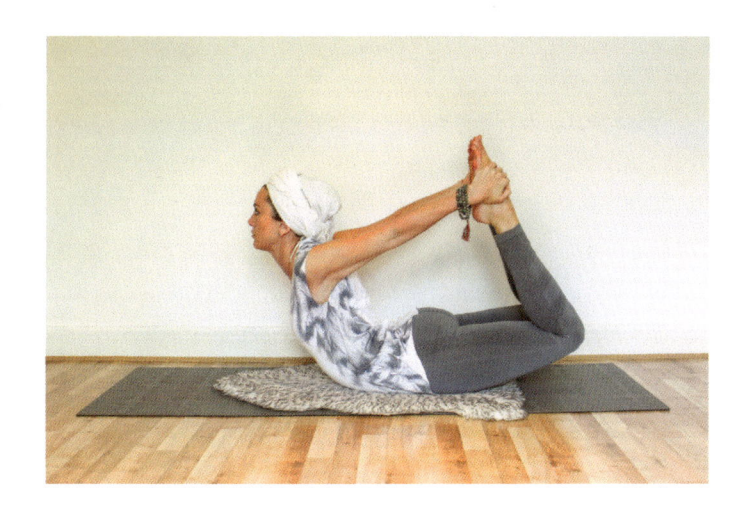

5. Rocking Bow Pose 1 Minute

Instructions: Lying on your stomach, reach back and take hold of the tops of the feet or ankles with the hands. Then push the shins away from the body whilst pulling with straight arms. Lift the chest and bring the head up and back. Ultimately, you want your thighs to lift off the ground. Now, keeping this position, start rocking back and forth on your stomach. Do what you can.

To end, inhale and arch up then exhale and relax.

Benefits: This opens the diaphragm and chest, energizes the sex nerve and is good for the pelvis, hips and spine.

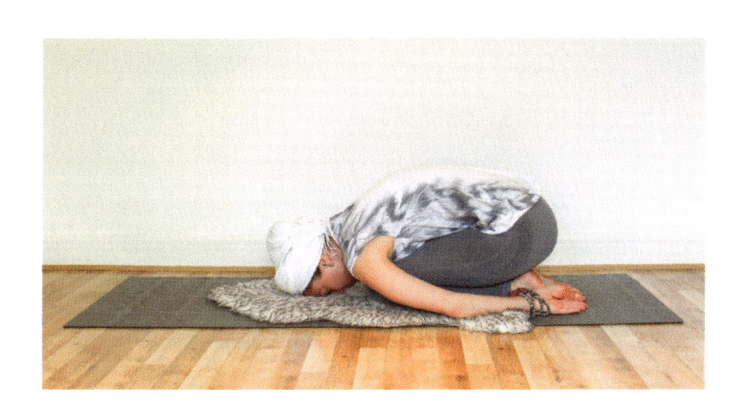

6. Baby Pose 1 Minute

Instructions: From your stomach, push back onto hands and knees and ease down to sit in your heels. Rest your forehead on the mat and bring your hands beside you. Relax.

Benefits: This calms the mind, elongates the lower back, opens the hips and is good for digestion.

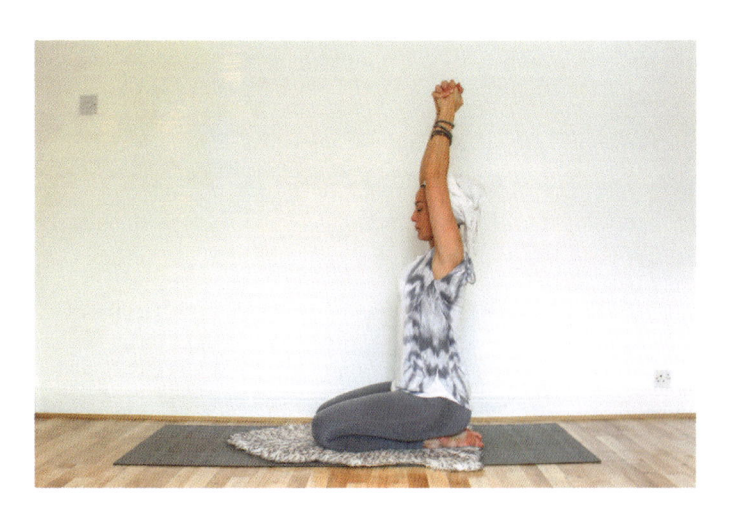

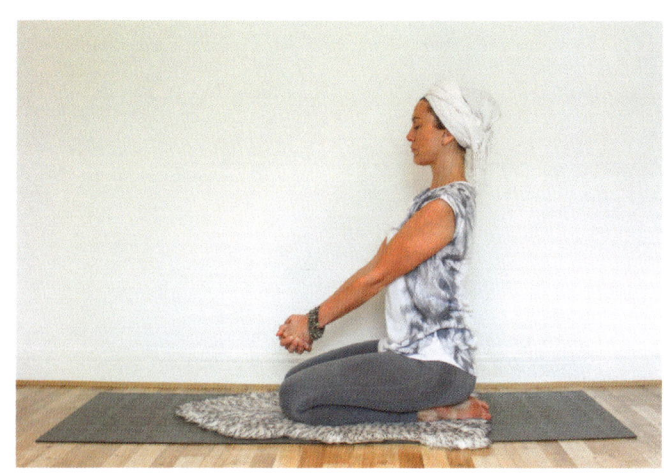

7. Wood Chops 1 Minute

Instructions: Sit up on the heels in Rock Pose (otherwise find a way to sit with your spine straight). Interlace your fingers in your lap, then inhale them up and exhale them down. Keep the arms straight.

Benefits: This loosens and strengthens the shoulders and opens the lungs.

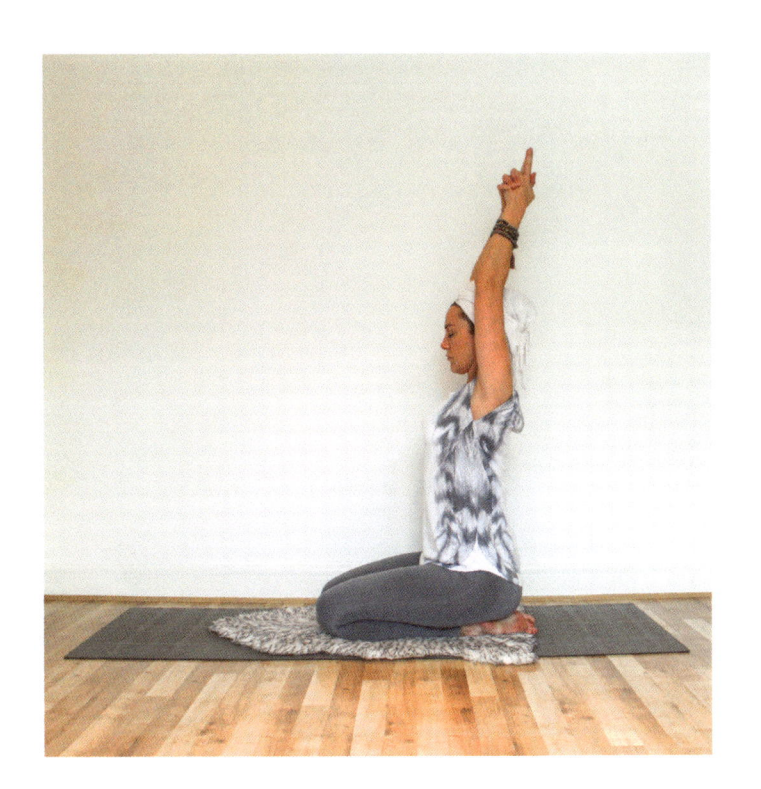

8. Sat Kriya 3 Minutes

Instructions: Sit in Rock Pose and interlace the fingers but keep the index fingers pointing up. Ladies, bring your left thumb over the right. Gent's, your right thumb comes over the left. Raise the arms straight up above the head but keep your shoulders relaxed. Chant 'Sat' (true) from the navel as you apply Mula Bandha and 'Nam' (name or identity) as you release the lock and your energy up to the Third Eye. To end, inhale, stretch up, apply Mula Bandha, exhale and relax. The breath will find its own way.

Benefits: This exercise is specifically designed to raise the Kundalini – your vital, life force. It also calms the nervous system and strengthens the entire sexual system, whilst channelling its natural flow of energy.

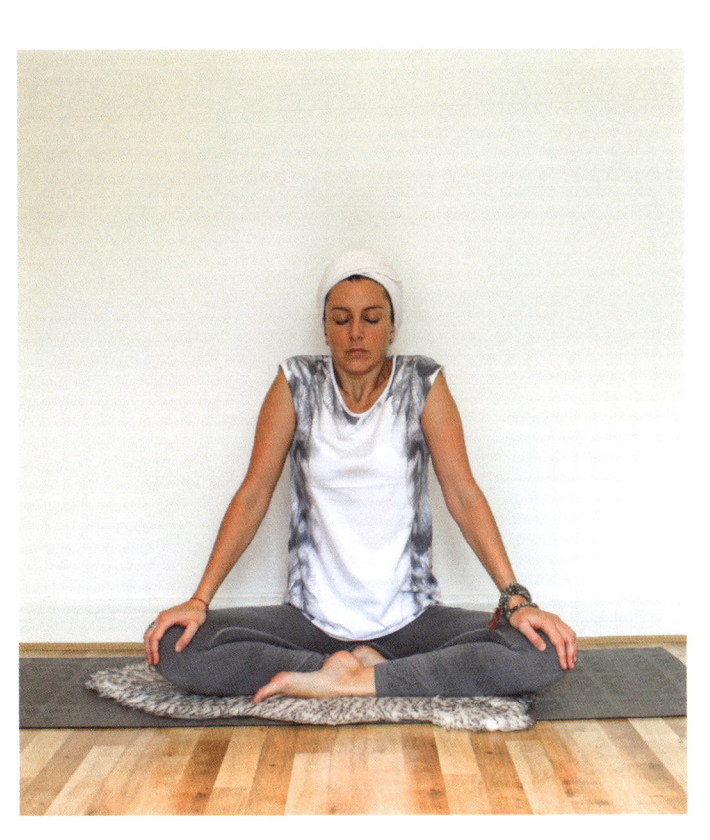

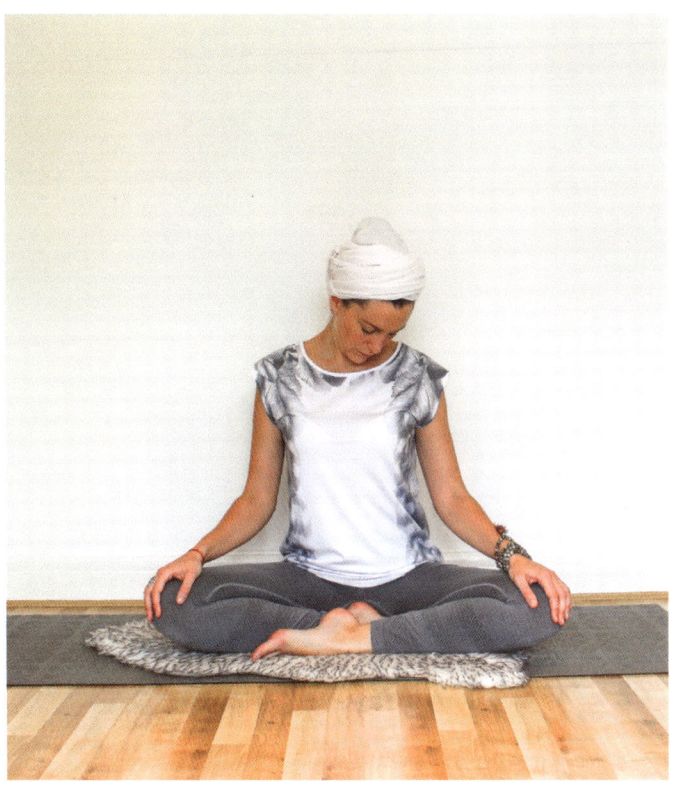

9. Head & Shoulder Rolls 6-8 Rolls in Each Direction

Instructions: Sitting with your hands on knees, begin rolling the shoulders forwards and up as you inhale and back around as you exhale. Then move to the neck, inhaling as you round forwards and exhaling as you round back.

Benefits: This opens the blood flow to the head, releases any tension in the neck and shoulders and rejuvenates the brain.

MEDITATION

SHABD KRIYA

POSITION

Sit with a straight spine and rest the hands in your lap, back of the right hand nestled in the pal of your left, thumb tips touching and facing forward. The eyes are nine tenths closed, focussed on the tip of the nose.

BREATH

Inhale in four equal parts, mentally chanting 'SaTaNaMa'. Then hold your breath for four mental repetitions of 'SaTaNaMa' (16 beats all together). Then exhale in two parts, mentally chanting 'Wahe Guru'.

MANTRA

Sa Ta Na Ma
Wahe Guru

DURATION

15 Minutes

TO END:

Inhale and hold the breath for 5-10 seconds then exhale and relax.

COMMENTS

This meditation helps you to relax, develop patience and become radiant. It regulates the breath into 22 beats. In Numerology, 11 is the number of Infinity and 22 symbolises mastery over the mental realm. This meditation, therefore, allows the mind an opportunity to connect with the neutral state of Infinity.

SaTaNaMa is the bij or seed mantra Sat Nam (True Name) broken down into syllables or the cycle of life — Infinity, Life, Death, Rebirth.

Wahe Guru is the ecstasy when you learn by shining light on your darkness.

#embodyyoursoulpurpose
@roisinallanakiernan

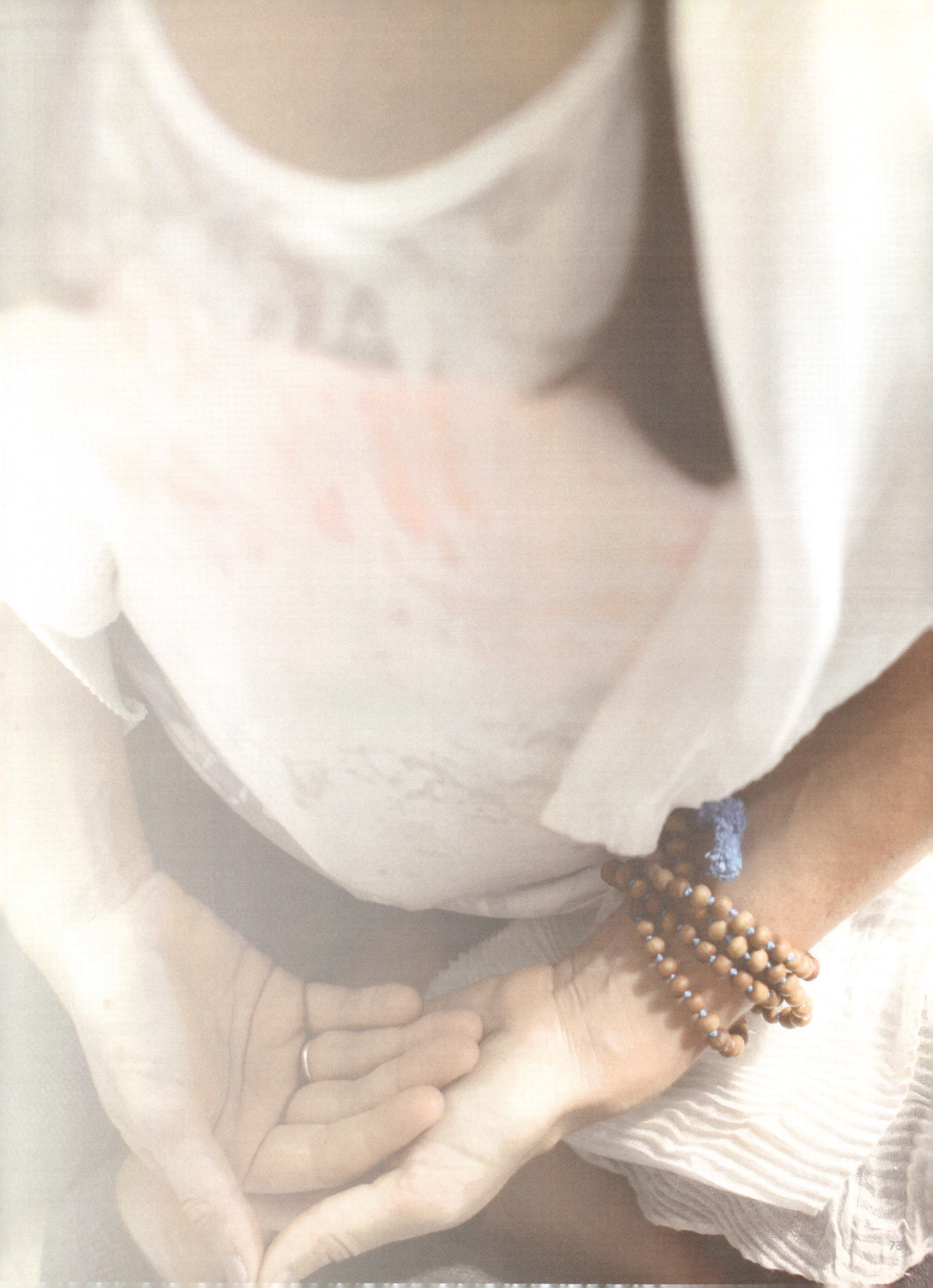

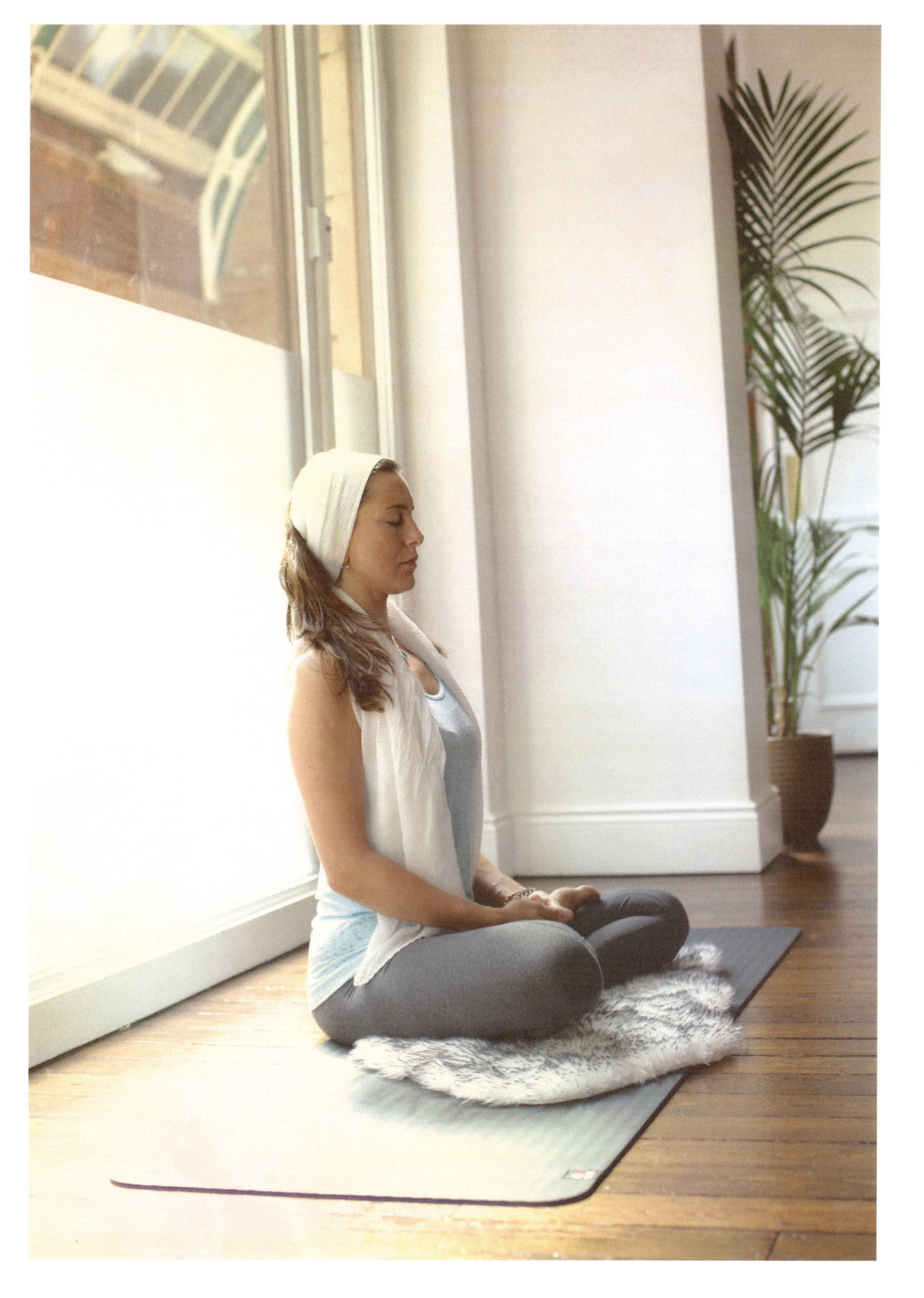

5

THE PHYSICAL BODY
COMMUNICATION INVOLVES LISTENING

Five is the half way point to ten – the bridge, or communicative link; the teacher. Are you participating fully – receiving all messages and responding in service, for others and yourself?

#embodyyoursoulpurpose

@roisinallanakiernan

THE PHYSICAL BODY
COMMUNICATION INVOLVES LISTENING

Understanding this fifth, Physical Body, might seem easy – you know your body, right? But do you know how you are using it? Are you even aware of your personal energy? Do you know – beyond the words you speak – how you are communicating? And how is your physical energy – is it balanced between doing and being, between giving and receiving?

Communication is key to the fifth, Physical Body. Communication with yourself – truly listening to your body and soul and responding in kind. And communication beyond words – the messages between your inner and outer self and between your physical body and another's.

Every aspect of life is experienced through the physical body. Yet it's easy to forget the miraculous nature of your body. It's easy to disregard the messages it's sending you too.

Through the physical your soul draws in people and situations that can help its journey. If you really listen during each situation or meeting you'll find that most will have a message for you. In this way you can use your physical body with wisdom to serve yourself and others.

A strong Physical Body offers the gift of teaching – an opportunity to relate and share tools for growth. A great teacher will intuitively receive the messages sent out through another's body and sensitively respond, at an appropriate communicative level, through their whole being. This talent requires great sensitivity, which equals mastery over the Physical Body.

This mastery over the Physical Body requires balance – between listening and speaking and between receiving and giving – in every moment. Are you receiving the messages you're being offered in order to help you move forward in life? Are you also carefully communicating the needs necessary for yours and others' growth? How you feel about your body must also be in balance - too much focus on the physical can show a disregard for the soul; not enough focus and the soul has no anchor.

Five marks the half way point to ten, which makes it the bridge – the communicative link (the Fifth Chakra also relates to the throat, which is all about communication). Being half-way denotes a point of transformation too, should you choose – an opportunity to sacrifice one state of being for another. It is through the physical body that we work through the karmas of our previous lifetimes and then transition into the next physical body and so on. It is also through five senses that your inner and outer selves communicate and you then communicate with another.

Your physical shape is reflective of where you're at in your life – how you feel on the inside is reflected on the outside. There is always a physical response to a thought too – negative thoughts will have an effect on the body, as will reactions to certain events. Feelings that you disregard will be held in the physical body and will eventually show through discomfort or illness. Of course you can work through such issues with the body – by stretching and being aware of aches and their causes; illnesses and their roots. The body can be our greatest teacher - if only we listen.

Paradoxically, it is also through the experience of polarities in the body that an existing sense of self is realised. In this way, you start to realise the part of you that cannot be fixed into time and space – the soul self or spirit; the invisible part of you. The infinite part of you that cannot be without the finite and yet existed before this physical life and will continue after. It is from this place of being that we can live moment by moment in balance, as a self that is and yet is not.

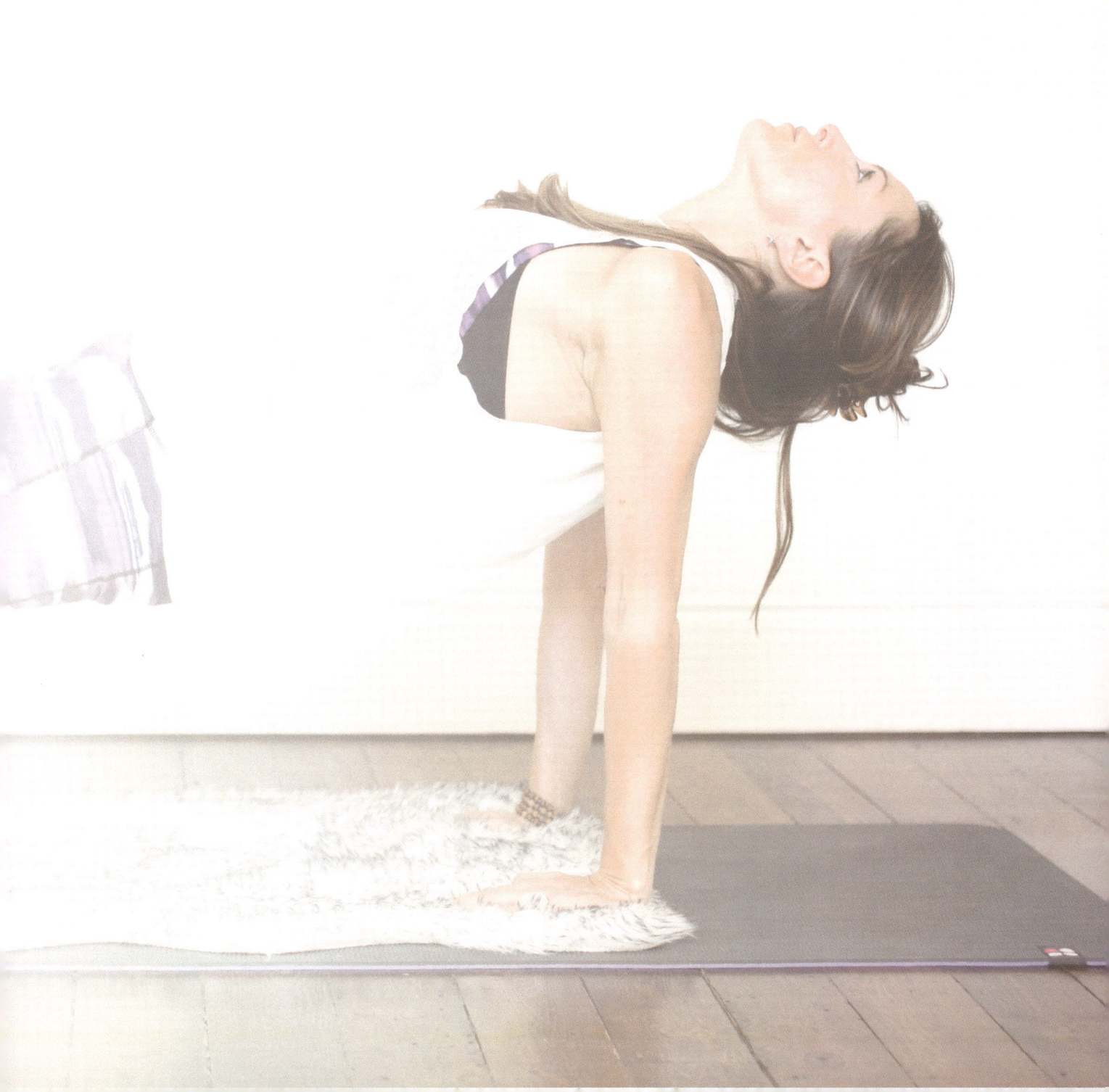

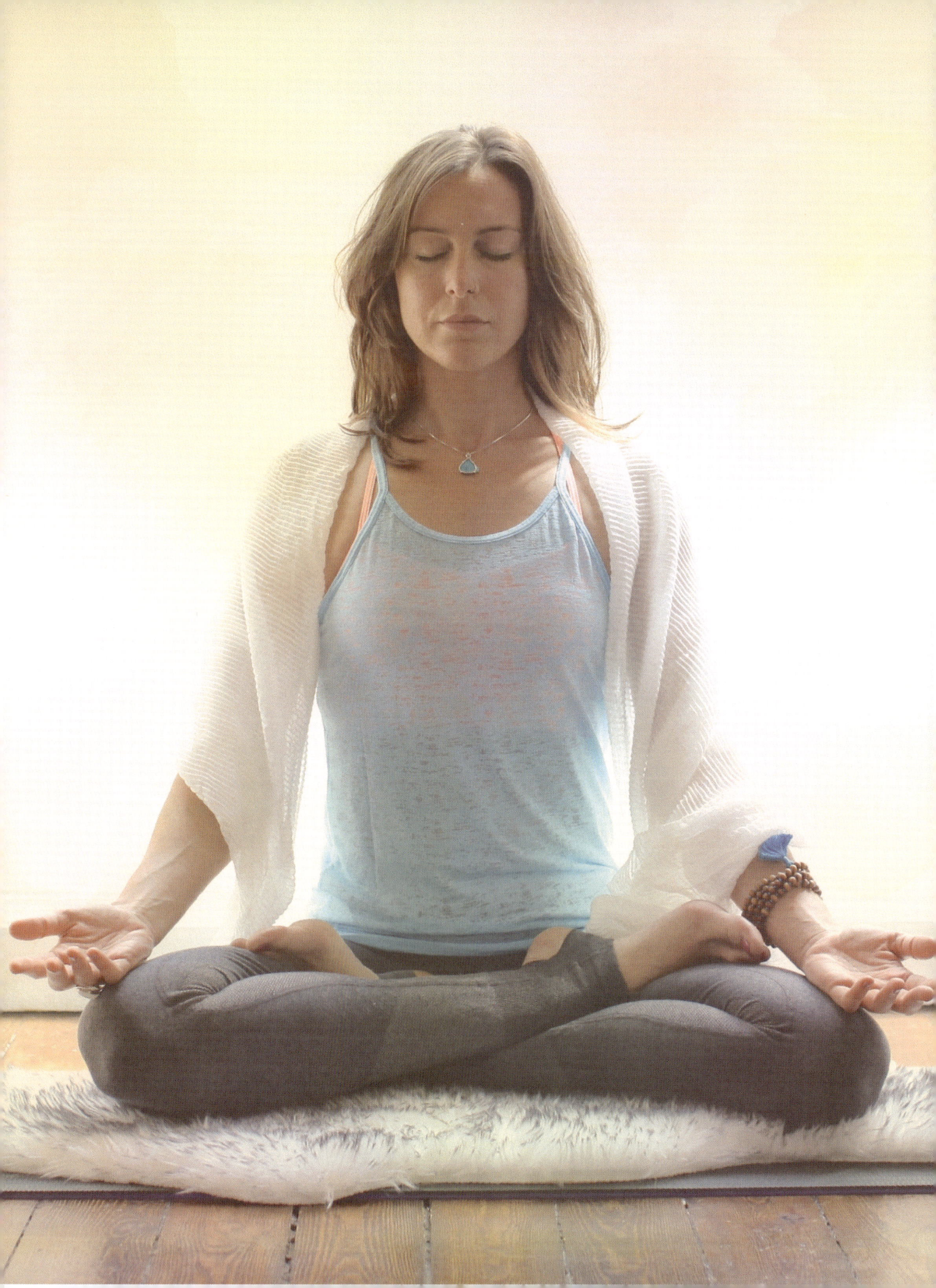

PRANAYAMA
BREATHING INTO YOUR TEN BODIES

POSITION & BREATH

Sitting with a straight spine, become aware of your breath – we're going to direct it through your Ten Bodies (you can use the visual Ten Bodies image on page 18 to guide you).

Starting with the Soul Body at the heart space, breathe long, deep breaths, picturing the breath as light being drawn in and out of the chest – allow it to fill, rise and fall with this light.

Then, draw the breath from the heart up to the left side of the brain, before drawing it over to the right and then, finally, into the middle (through the Soul, Negative, Positive and Neutral Minds). Your breath will feel like it's doing a little loop – down to heart, up to left brain, right and then middle.

Continue with this loop of light and then draw it through the rest of the phyiscal body – filling each part with light. Take your time. Breathe light and space into every organ and limb and across every inch of skin.

Then breathe out into the 6th, 7th, 8th, 9th and 10th Bodies beyond the 5th Physical Body. Allow yourself to feel the space you occupy beyond the physical. Expand. Feel your vastness.

DURATION

3-22 Minutes

Teachers, 11 minutes would be a great amount of time to add this into the beginning of your class. Guide your students through each section or body, so they have enough time to work through each. Once they understand, 3 minutes at the beginning of a class would suffice. Over 11 minutes would turn this into a deep meditation.

TO END

After exhaling, simply allow the breath to return to its natural rhythm and take a moment to feel into each of The Ten Bodies, especially the energetic, lesser known aspects of the self.

COMMENTS

This is a great tool to build your awareness of The Ten Bodies. It also expands your sense of self beyond the physical – allowing you to feel into the space you occupy around the body.

NB: This is my own breathing exercise, which I've developed to connect with The Ten Bodies. It is not Yogi Bhajan's teachings.

#embodyyoursoulpurpose
@roisinallanakiernan

KRIYA
FOUNDATION FOR INFINITY

This set works primarily on the pelvic region, setting your foundation in the physical, so the Infinite can be accessed in meditation. Physiologically the pelvis acts as the point of balance for your torso and lower foundation on Earth. The female pelvis is especially delicate and can misalign, leading to sciatica and menstrual irregularities. Pelvis misalignment in men can lead to conditions such as impotency. This set works to strengthen the pelvic area.

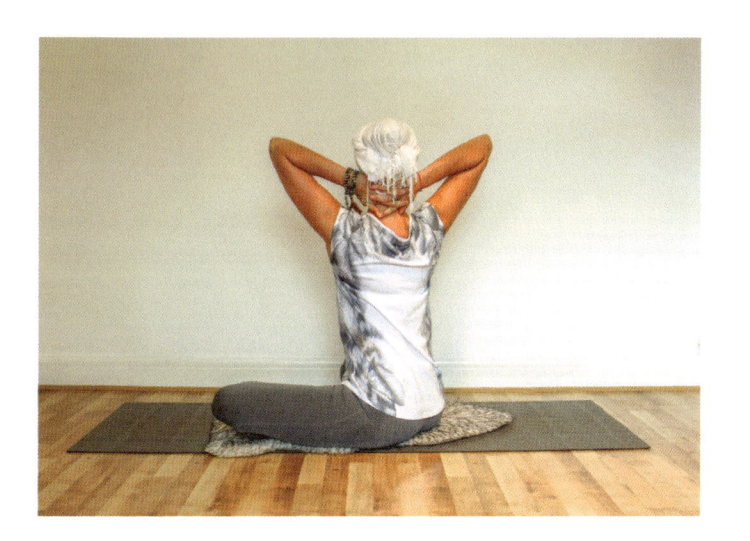

1. Spinal Twist Variation   3 Minutes

Instructions: Sit with your spine straight and interlock the hands behind the neck at the hairline under any loose hair. Holding this position, inhale and twist to the left, then exhale and twist to the right. Continue at a medium pace.

Benefits: This works to open the shoulders and upper back. The twist adds a detoxifying process too.

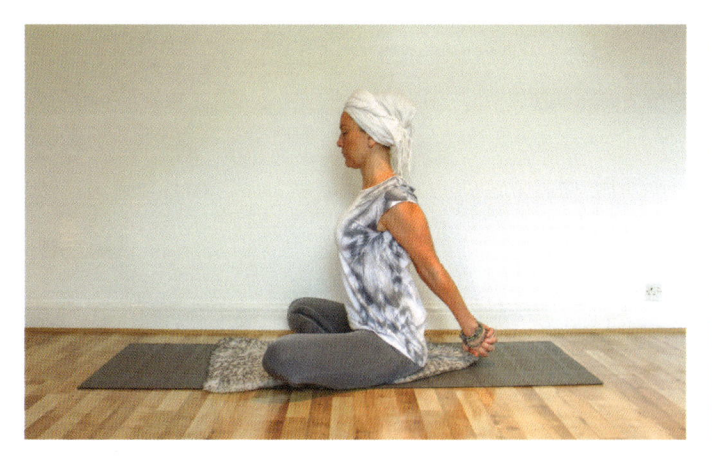

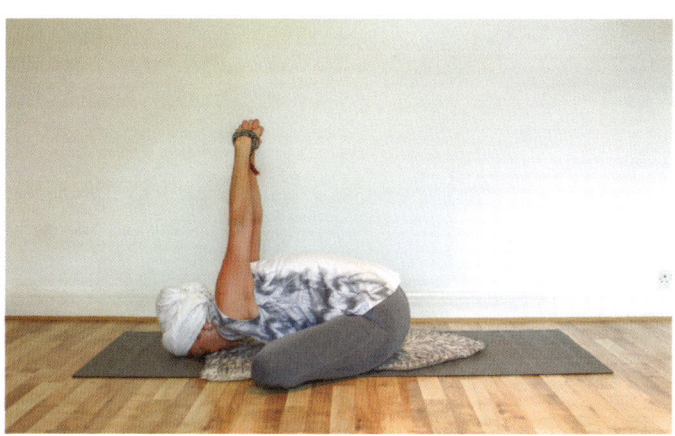

2. Yoga Mudra with Breath of Fire   2 Minutes

Instructions: Sit with a straight spine and interlock your fingers behind the back. Then begin Breath of Fire and alternate between this posture and Yoga Mudra – forehead to the mat and hands (still interlocked behind the back) raised with straight arms. Move at a steady pace, coordinating your movements with the breath.

Benefits: Breath of Fire is rejuvenating in itself. The arm position also works to open the chest and shoulders.

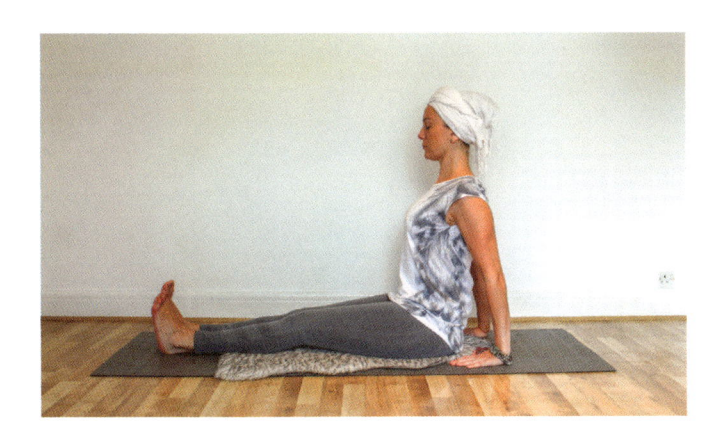

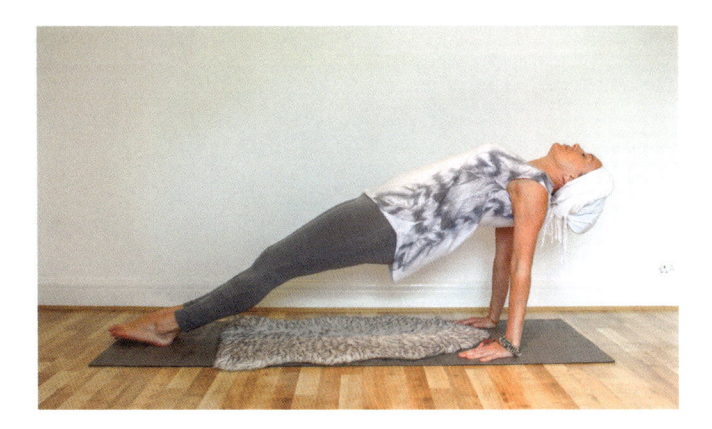

3. Back Platform Flow with Breath of Fire   1-5 Minutes

Instructions: Sit with your legs straight out and your hands flat on the floor by your sides, fingers pointing forwards. Then, as you inhale, lift the hips with the legs straight, so the whole body lifts up, supported by the hands and feet. Lower your head back, if you can. (An alternative for those with a weaker core or lower back, would be to keep the feet flat on the floor and bend the knees while lifting the hips.) From Back Platform, begin Breath of Fire and move between the start point (bottom down) and up, coordinating the movement with the breath.

Benefits: This increases the strength and flexibility of the pelvic area and releases the pelvis if it's locked.

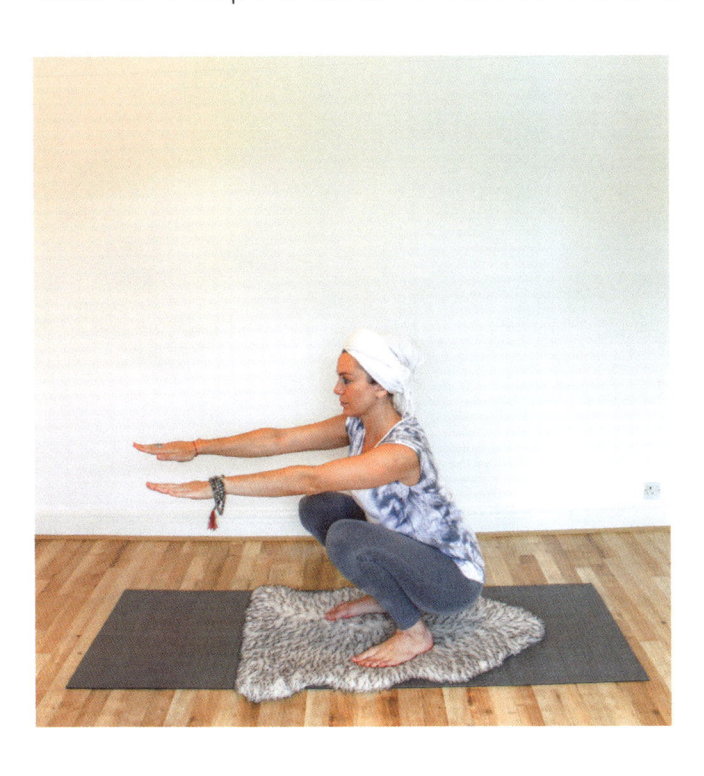

4. Crow Pose Squats   26 Times

Instructions: Stand with your feet turned out to the sides, then sit down into your haunches, bending the knees but keeping the feet flat. Then bring your hands straight out in front of you, palms facing down. Inhale and stand up, exhale and squat down into Crow Pose.

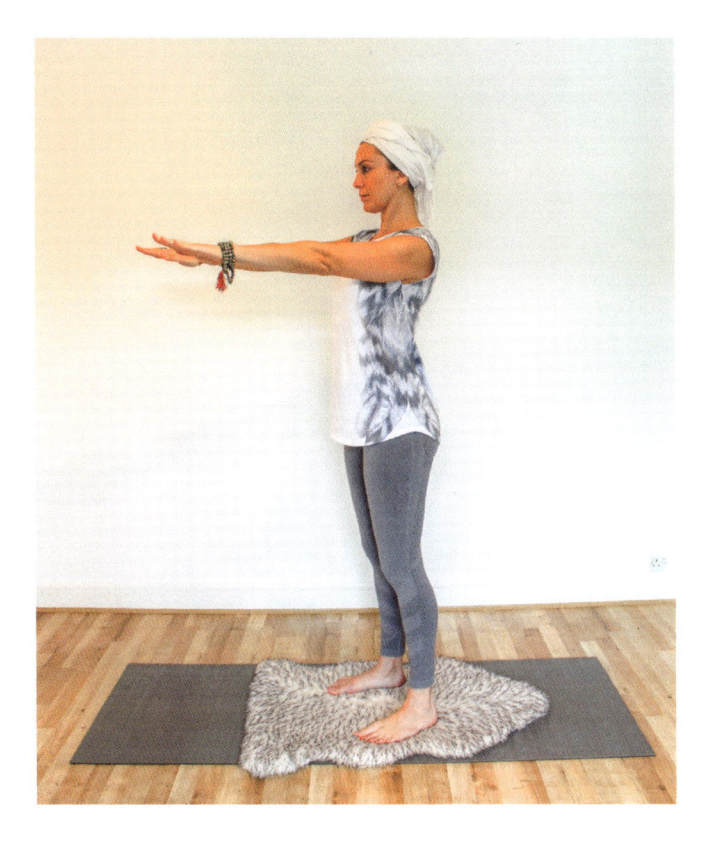

Benefits: These are good for your circulation and digestion. They also build muscles throughout the body and improve knee flexibility.

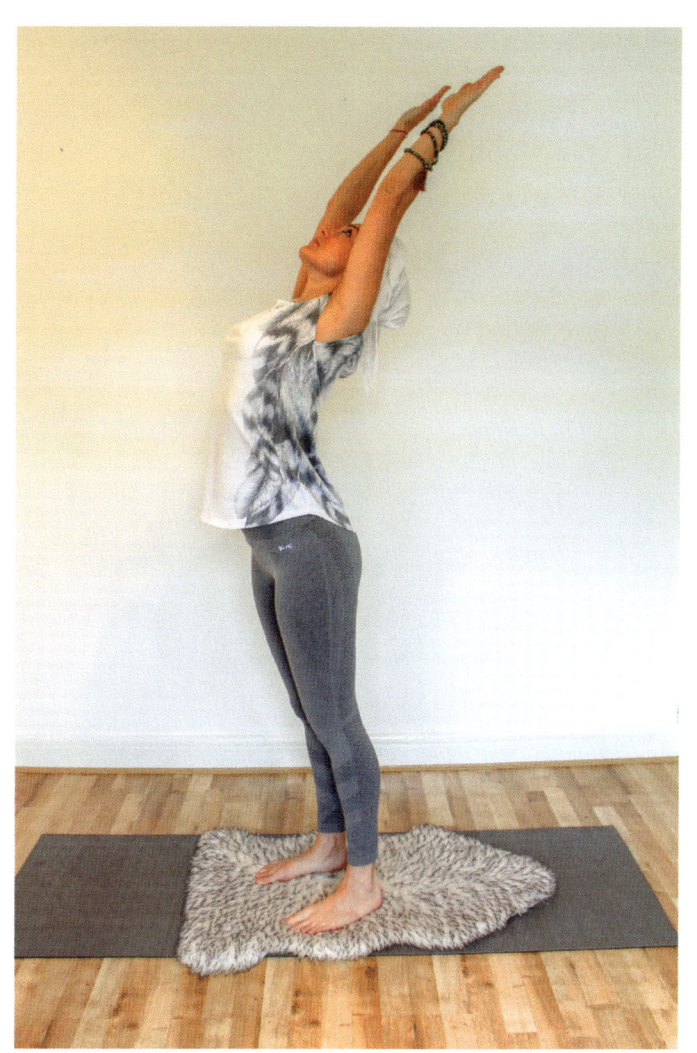

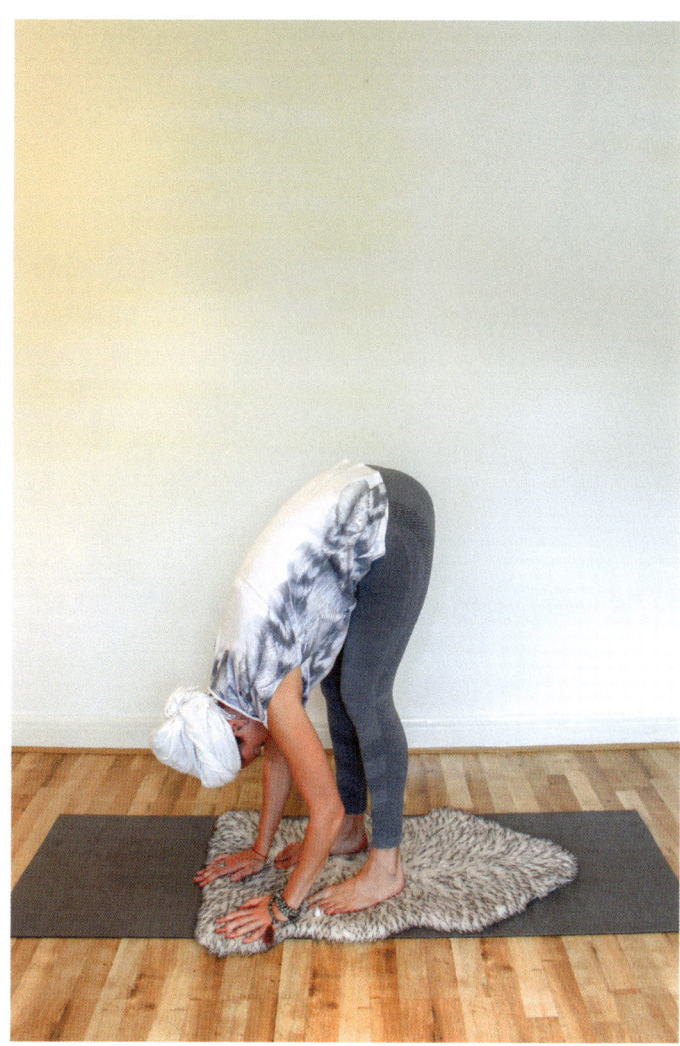

5. Front Bends 1-5 Minutes

Instructions: Stand with your legs shoulder width apart and extend the arms above the head, palms facing forward. Inhale and stretch back as far as possible (being careful of your lower back as you do) then exhale and fold forward over the legs.

Benefits: This revitalises the brain, gets the spinal fluid moving and stretches the hamstrings, calves and hips.

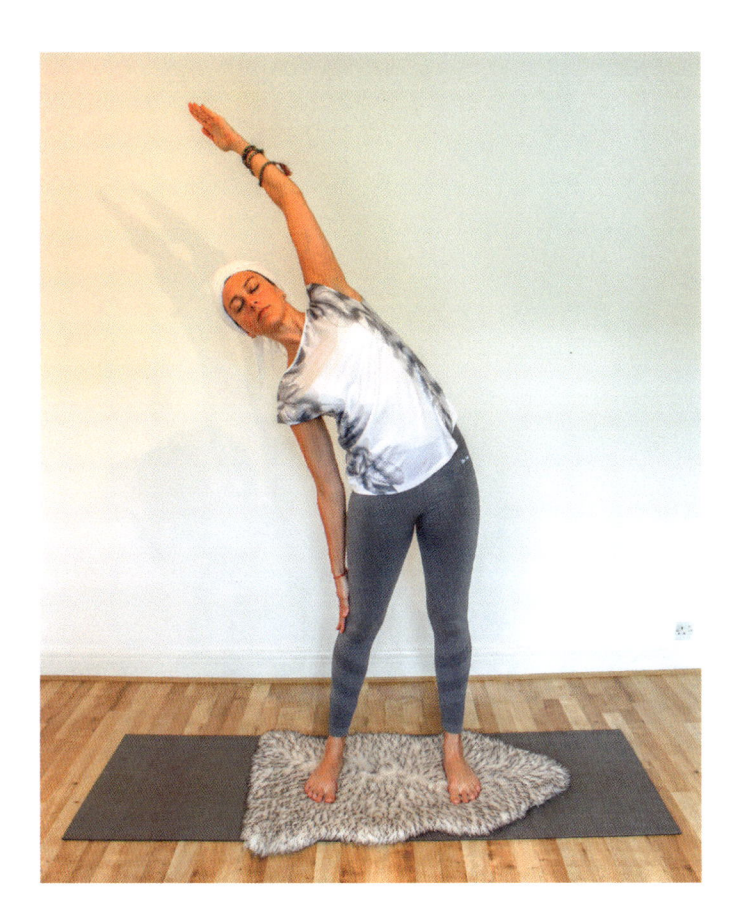

6. Side Stretch   26 Times

Instructions: Standing straight, inhale as you bend over to the left, bringing your right arm over to deepen the stretch. Then exhale to your right, with the left arm reaching over. Make sure the stretch comes from your side – keep the shoulders squared.

Benefits: This is a great exercise for people who sit at desks for long periods of time, because it stretches the Quadratus Lumborum (QL), which can become short and stiff if left unused, leading to lower back injuries.

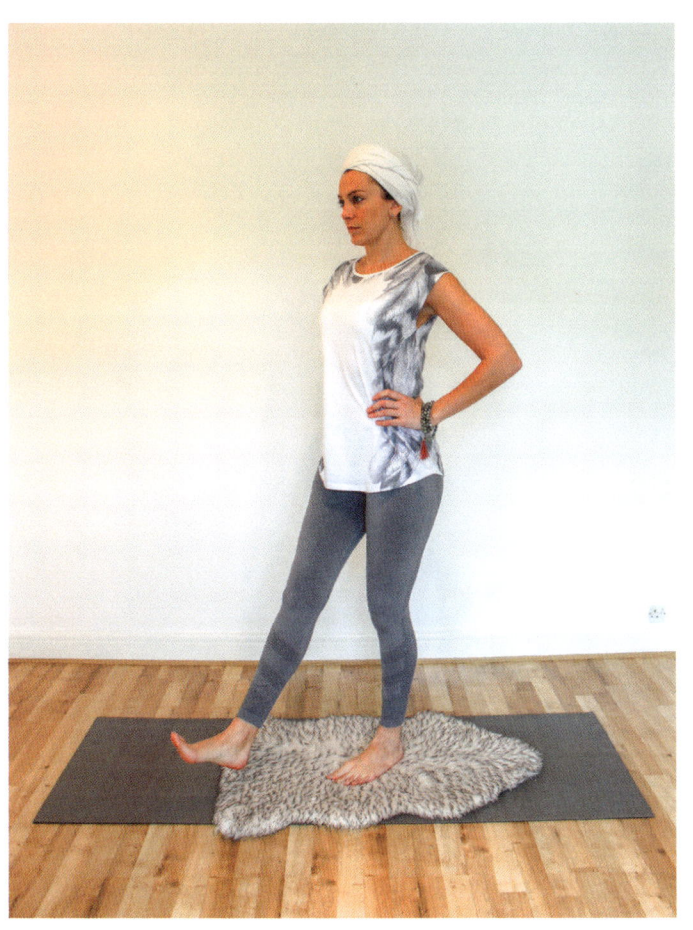

7. Rhythmic Kick with Har Mantra

3 Minutes

Instructions: Stand with your hands on your hips and, keeping the legs straight, alternatively kick your feet, chanting Har (meaning We or God or the Universe) from the navel each time. The Tantric Har recording works well with this.

Benefits: I like to explain this as kicking off everything that's holding you back from connecting with the infinite/all. It literally kicks your will-power into gear and balances it so that your will is in line with that of the divine's.

NB: The following meditation is part of this kriya. Please continue on to the meditation to complete the kriya.

MEDITATION

FOR THE TENTH GATE: TO EXPERIENCE YOUR BOUNDLESSNESS

POSITION

Sit with a straight spine and relax the hands in your lap (right hand on top of left) with the palms facing up, pads of the thumbs touching.

Roll your eyes up to look out of the top of the head – to your Tenth Gate (Crown Chakra). Mentally chant the mantra Har Har as you pull the navel in. Then, holding the navel in, press the tip of the tongue against the roof of the mouth and mentally say Mukanday.

MANTRA

Har Har
Mukanday

BREATH

The breath will find its own rhythm.

DURATION

11 - 13 Minutes

COMMENTS

Allow yourself to surrender into the vastness of being. Feel yourself expand beyond time and space, into a realm of total peace and joy.

Har is another word for We or God or the Divine Universe. Mukanday is the Har within the individual – it's the infinite, liberating aspect of the self. This mantra works to remove fear and turns challenges into opportunities, liberating a person from their blocks.

#embodyyoursoulpurpose
@roisinallanakiernan

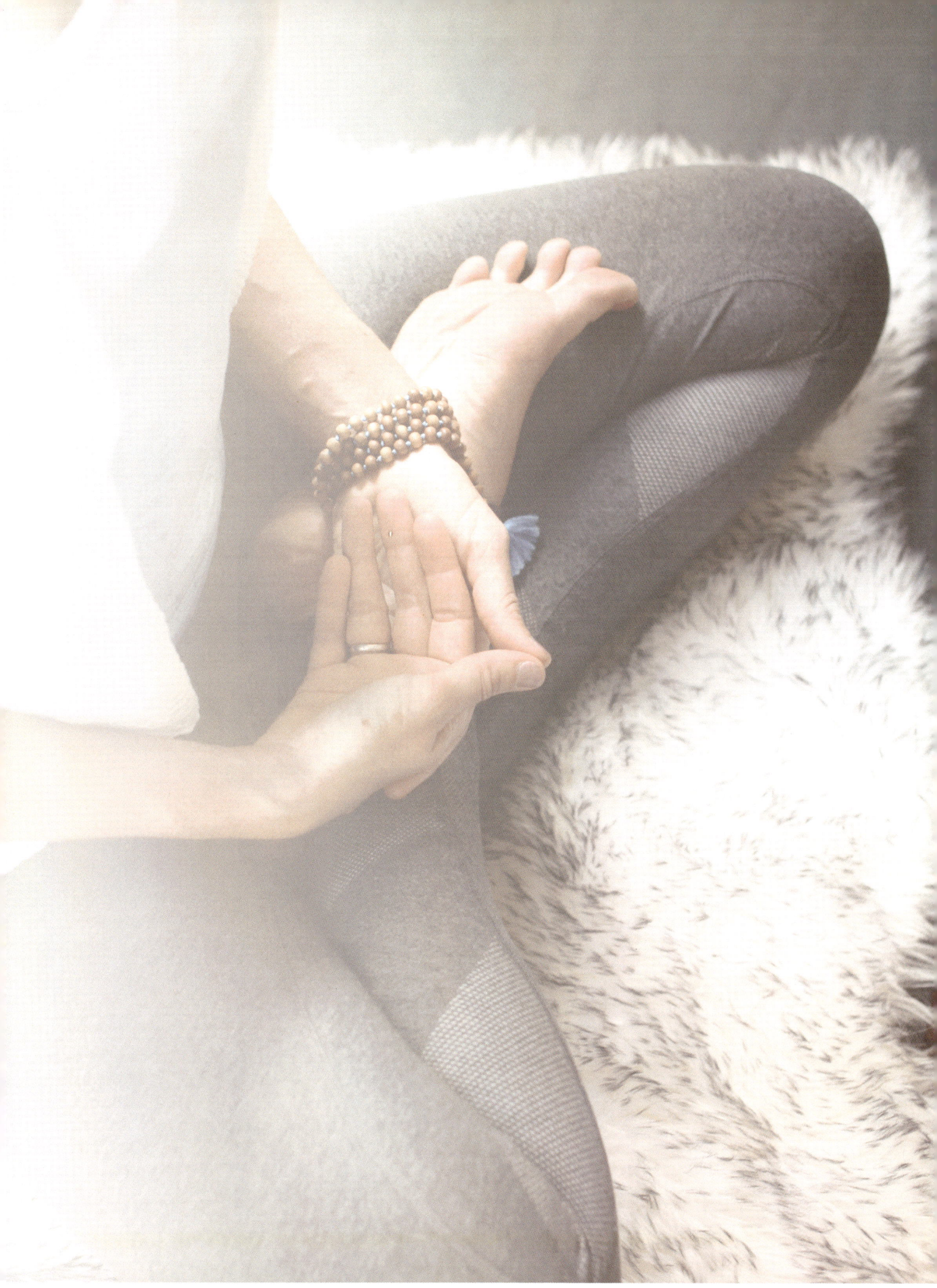

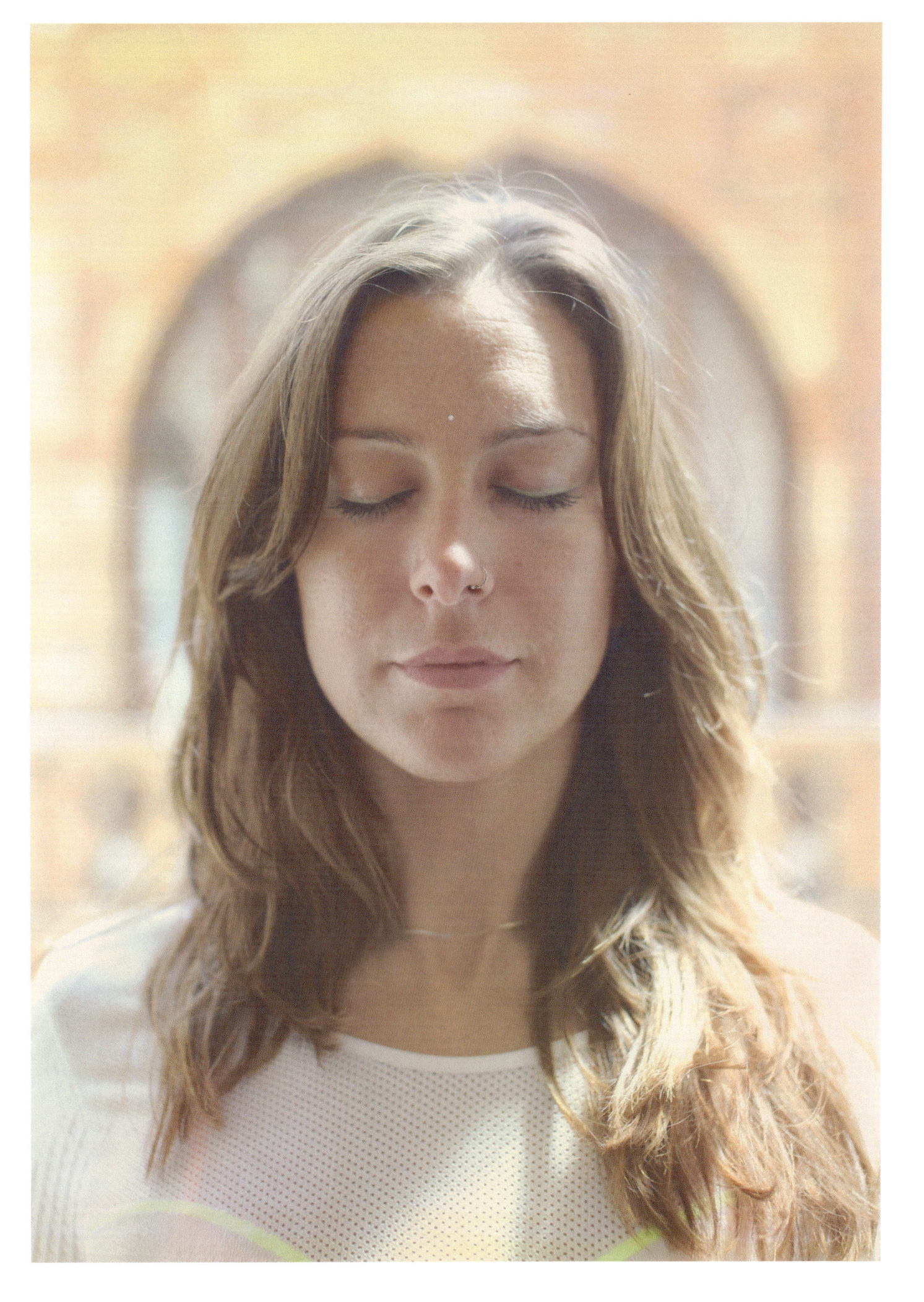

6

THE ARCLINE

WORRIER OR WARRIOR

This is your halo, symbolised by a sword, which can be pointed at you (worry) or away from you (warrior). What you put out, or point towards yourself, all depends on you. Strengthen the subtleties of this body to alert and guide you with integrity.

#embodyyoursoulpurpose

@roisinallanakiernan

THE ARCLINE
WORRIER OR WARRIOR

You know those images of Gods and Saints with a Halo (a luminous ring of light) around their heads? Well, you also have a Halo, or an Arcline. In fact, women have two – one around the head and another from nipple to nipple. They're symbolised by the sword.

The Arcline is like a double-edged sword – it can be pointed towards you (like a wOrrier) or away from you (like a wArrior). For the Arcline is about projection and, therefore, what you put out, or point towards yourself, all depends on you.

The Sixth Body relates to the Sixth Chakra – the Ajna or Third Eye – the seat of your intuition. So there's a subtlety involved – there's a reaching out to touch the world in a way that utilises all the senses, that listens to the body's guidance and wise, inner voice. When you really listen then you can predict, or intuit, the immediate future – you can be a warrior in the world, feeling your way.

The alternative of this warrior state is a worrier – someone who's scared of this natural sensitivity; who talks or keeps silent out of fear; who chooses to agree with another and go against their inner wisdom; who chooses to listen instead to the chatter of the mind.

Just like its symbol of the sword, the Arcline has a protective and projective nature. When strong it will work like an invisible shield, alerting you to dangers and guiding you to take the path best suited to your growth. When weak you're blinded to the signs or stuck in fear and can open yourself to danger, accidents or illness. Ultimately, it's your choice to listen to yourself – to protect or project yourself. In this respect, the projection of your Arcline corresponds with your integrity.

Living your truth isn't easy – it takes listening to that inner wisdom (that intuition) and choosing to act on it (projecting yourself with integrity) in every moment, without being fixed on the outcome. You have to know yourself - accept, understand and integrate your light and shadow self. When this takes shape, though, wow – then you start to create your reality with your projection.

When you have faith that your inner wisdom is correct and you let go of anything beyond the moment - when you work intuitively and with integrity - from a place of truth, then life blossoms gracefully. You also recognise the balance between your will and divine will.

The Arcline (or Halo) brings the left and right hemispheres of the brain into balance (our Protective/Negative and Projective/Positive Bodies) and then harnesses a meditative mental state (Neutral Mind). From this neutral state we feel more compassionately and act from a place of truth and justice. Then, in the Sixth Body (Arcline/Halo) your choice-making process starts to come from the spirit-mind. You can picture it – the glowing Halo, holding the left and right sides of the brain together, harnessing that neutral mind state and beaming your spirit/soul self through into being. Women can have extra sensitivity of being or beaming from their second Arcline or Halo, from nipple to nipple.

89

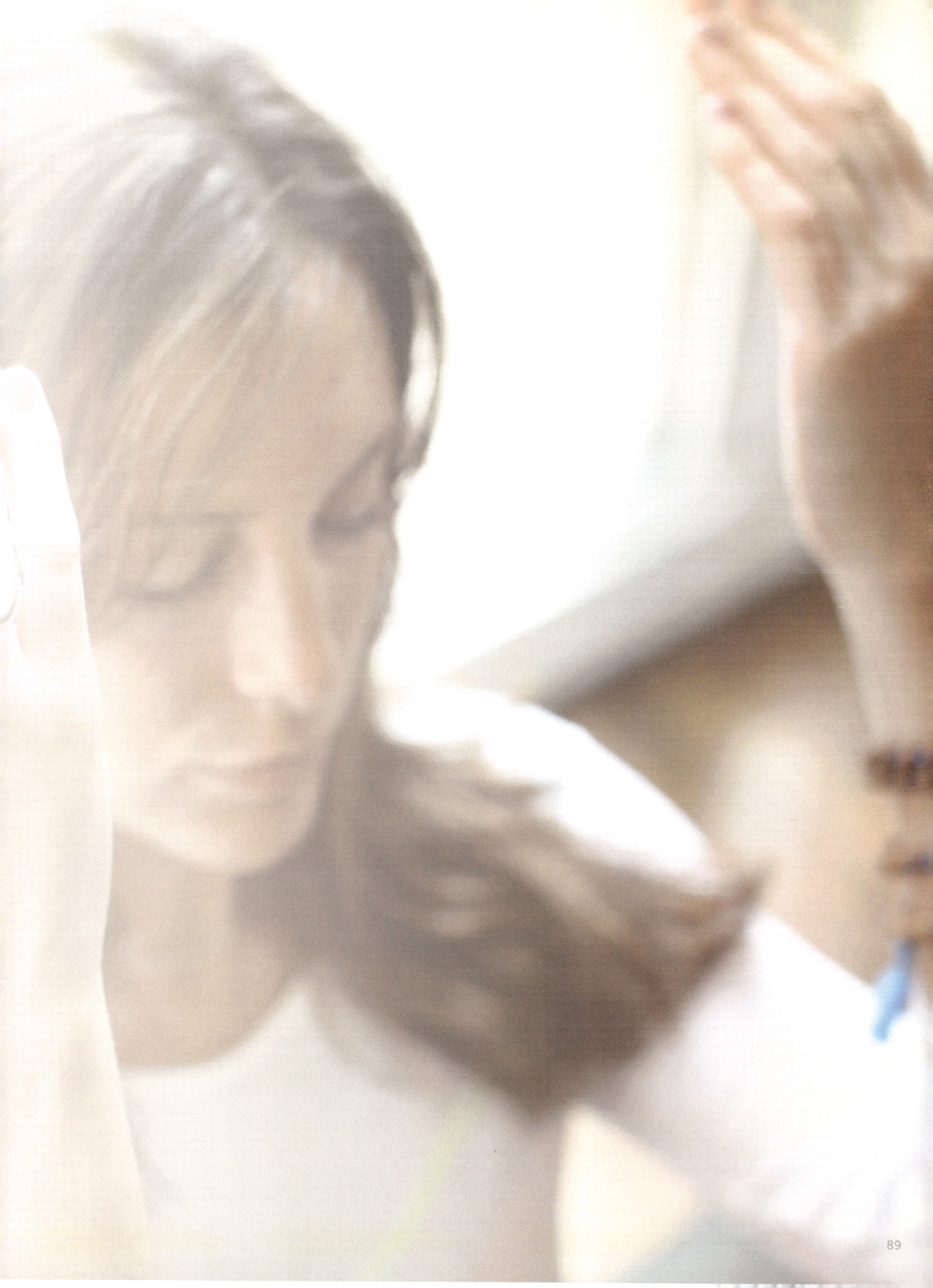

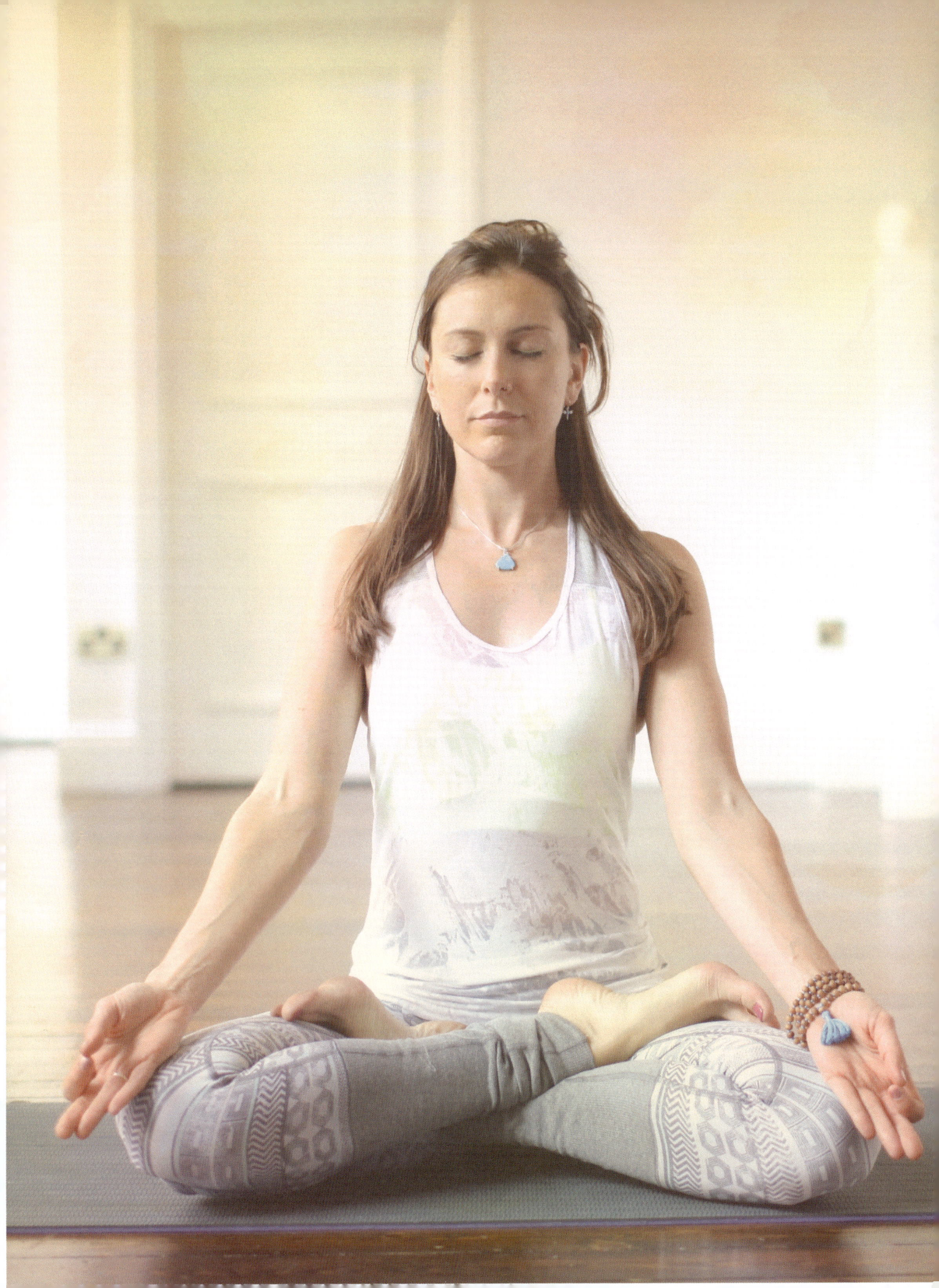

PRANAYAMA

DHRIB DHRISHTI LOCHINA KARMA, MEDITATION FOR INSPIRING TRUTHFUL, DEEPLY PENETRATING SPEECH

POSITION

Sitting with a tall spine, bring your hands into Gyan Mudra (index fingers touching thumbs) and place them in an active position, with the arms straight and your palms facing out. Then lock the edges of your front teeth together – you might need to move the whole of your lower jaw to do this.

The tongue touches the upper palate in a relaxed way. Gently focus your eyes on the tip of your nose.

Holding this position, mentally project the mantra 'Sa Ta Na Ma' out from your Third Eye. Create a powerful projection and let the rhythm find an internal harmony.

MANTRA

Sa Ta Na Ma

BREATH

The breath will find its own flow.

DURATION

15 - 31 Minutes

To master this meditation, you can slowly build your time to 1.5 hours at a sitting.

TO END

After an exhale, relax the position and send out blessings for peace.

COMMENTS

Sa Ta Na Ma is known as a Bij (seed) mantra and is designed to bring you in line with your destiny. It represents the cycle of life – Infinity, Life, Death, Rebirth / Sa, Ta, Na Ma – and makes up Sat Nam (True Name). Together with the position, this meditation works to enhance your awareness in thought and action. Your words will gain the power to penetrate deeply – they'll inspire and offer truth in any situation.

Full moons are an especially potent time to practise this meditation.

#embodyyoursoulpurpose
@roisinallanakiernan

KRIYA

ADJUST YOUR FLOW WITH THE FOUR U'S

This set invigorates you by adjusting your Pranic Body (the breath) with your Auric Body (your baggage) in direct contact with your arcline (your projection). Each of the following positions can be held for a minimum of three minutes, just make sure you hold each for the same amount of time. Try not to move at all once you're in these positions and make sure you have a good relaxation afterwards.

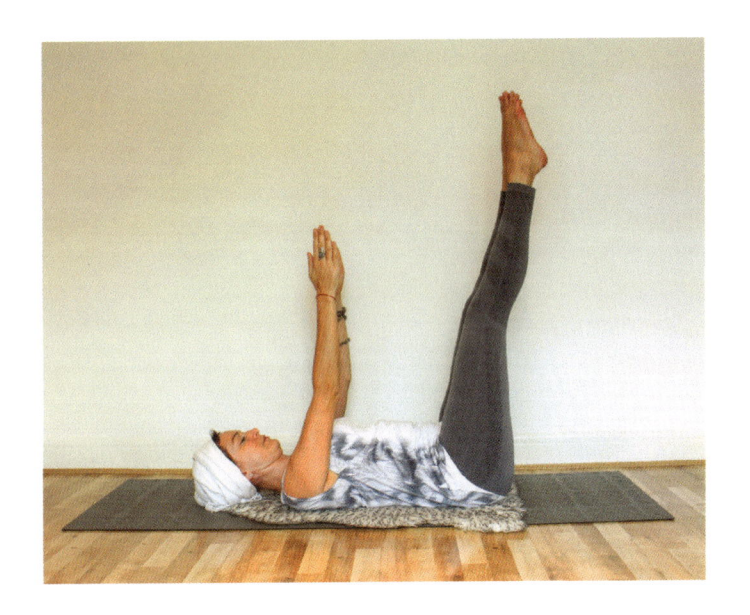

U No. 1   11 Minutes

Instructions: Lie on your back, raise your legs up to 90 degrees then bring your arms straight up from the shoulders too. Your legs are together, knees as straight as possible. The elbows remain straight too.

Benefits: "In this position, think about what good you have done since you arrived on Earth – bring your action-oriented ability in line with your beautiful intelligence. We are working, without movement, to move the 'chi' (energy) in this kriya. Stay still in this position – the energy will move itself." – Yogi Bhajan

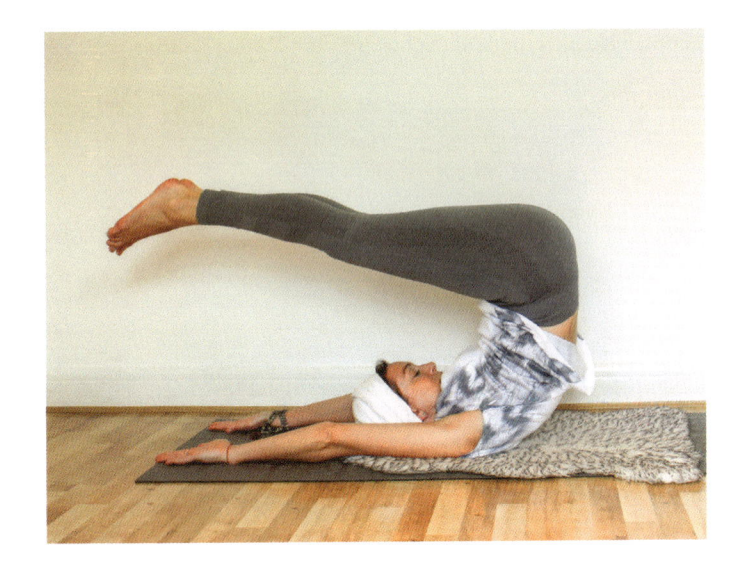

U No. 2   11 Minutes

Instructions: Remain on your back but bring your hands straight up over your head to the ground. Then raise your lower body up into a modified half Plow Pose, with your legs straight over the head but parallel to the ground. Keep your weight in your shoulders.

Benefits: Simply be; simply let the energy flow.

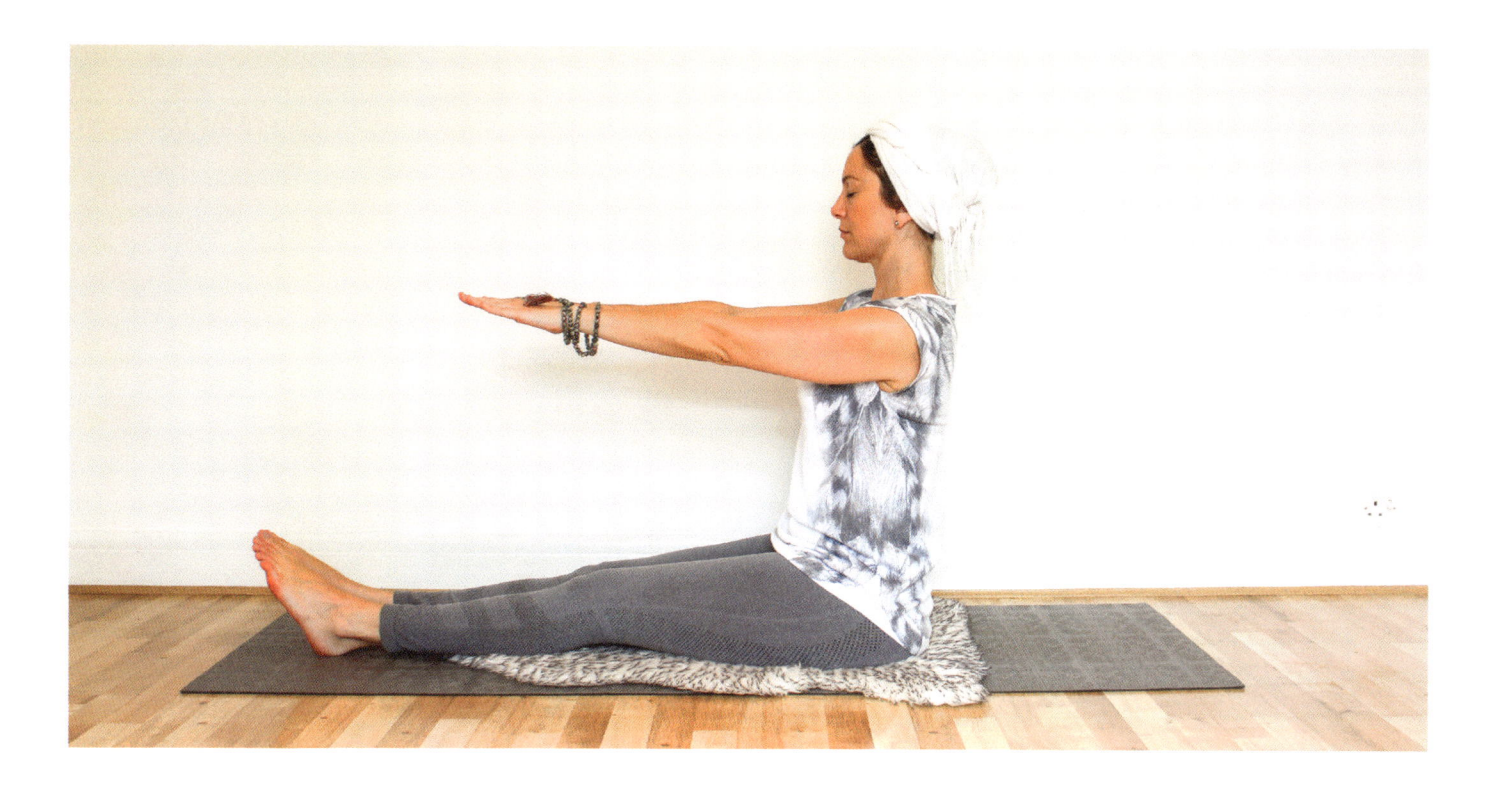

U No. 3 **11 Minutes**

Instructions: Sitting up now, stretch your legs out in front (hip distance apart) and put your hands straight out, so they're held directly above the legs. Keep your back straight.

Benefits: "As the energy moves, you might feel pain or uncomfortability in this position. This is the pressure of the muscles adjusting themselves. Try to keep your posture perfect – let it do the work." – Yogi Bhajan

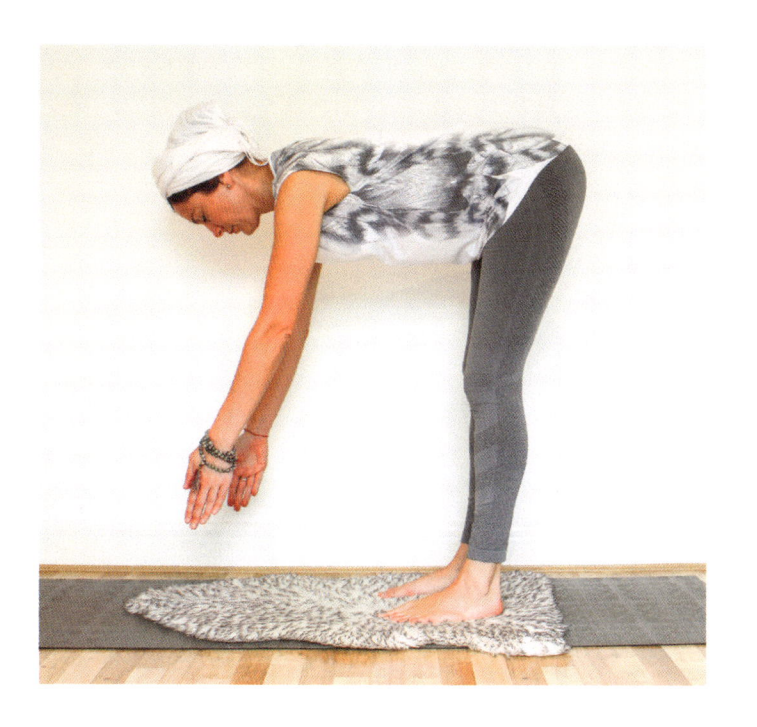

U No. 4 **11 Minutes**

Instructions: Standing, bend over at the waist so your torso is held parallel to the ground. Keep the back and neck straight and let your arms hang loosely down to the ground.

Benefits: "Don't bend down to the toes – keep the firm 'U' shape. It will set 'u' up." – Yogi Bhajan

MEDITATION

FOR THE ARCLINE AND TO CLEAR THE KARMAS

POSITION

Sit with a straight spine, bend your elbows and bring your hands out in front of you, palms slightly cupped a few inches above the knees.

As you inhale, bring the hands up and stretch them as far as you can back over the head. Imagine you're scooping water and throwing it through your Arcline – use a flick of the wrists to really get that washing feel. Bring the hands back down on the exhale and begin again on the inhale.

The movement is smooth and gracefully flows along with the lyrics and rhythm of the mantra music – 'Wahe Guru, Wahe Guru, Wahe Guru, Wahe Jio'. On each 'Wahe Guru' and on the 'Wahe Jio', do a full scoop up and back.

The eyes are closed.

MANTRA

Wahe Guru
Wahe Guru
Wahe Guru
Wahe Jio

DURATION

31 Minutes
One cycle of the mantra takes about 8-10 seconds.

TO END

Inhale and stretch your hands up and back as far as possible. Hold for 10-15 seconds then exhale. Repeat 3 times. And relax.

COMMENTS

This meditation will help you to experience what Wahe Guru actually means. Remember, the power of Infinity is not outside of you – it is in you. When 'I' and Infinity create impact then you'll become totally divine. Until the 'I and I' connect, you'll remain locked in duality, which keeps you away from reality and causes suffering.

Find a recording of this mantra music that you enjoy and let yourself really connect - clear the karmas of past generations and lives and reconnect with the Infinite.

There is a delicious Arcline meditation that's specifically for women - Meditation To Realise Your Power. It works to clear the heart's web or connections and increase the awareness of your energy's ability. Please see my YouTube channel for more information - access via my website www.roisinallanakiernan.com

#embodyyoursoulpurpose
@roisinallanakiernan

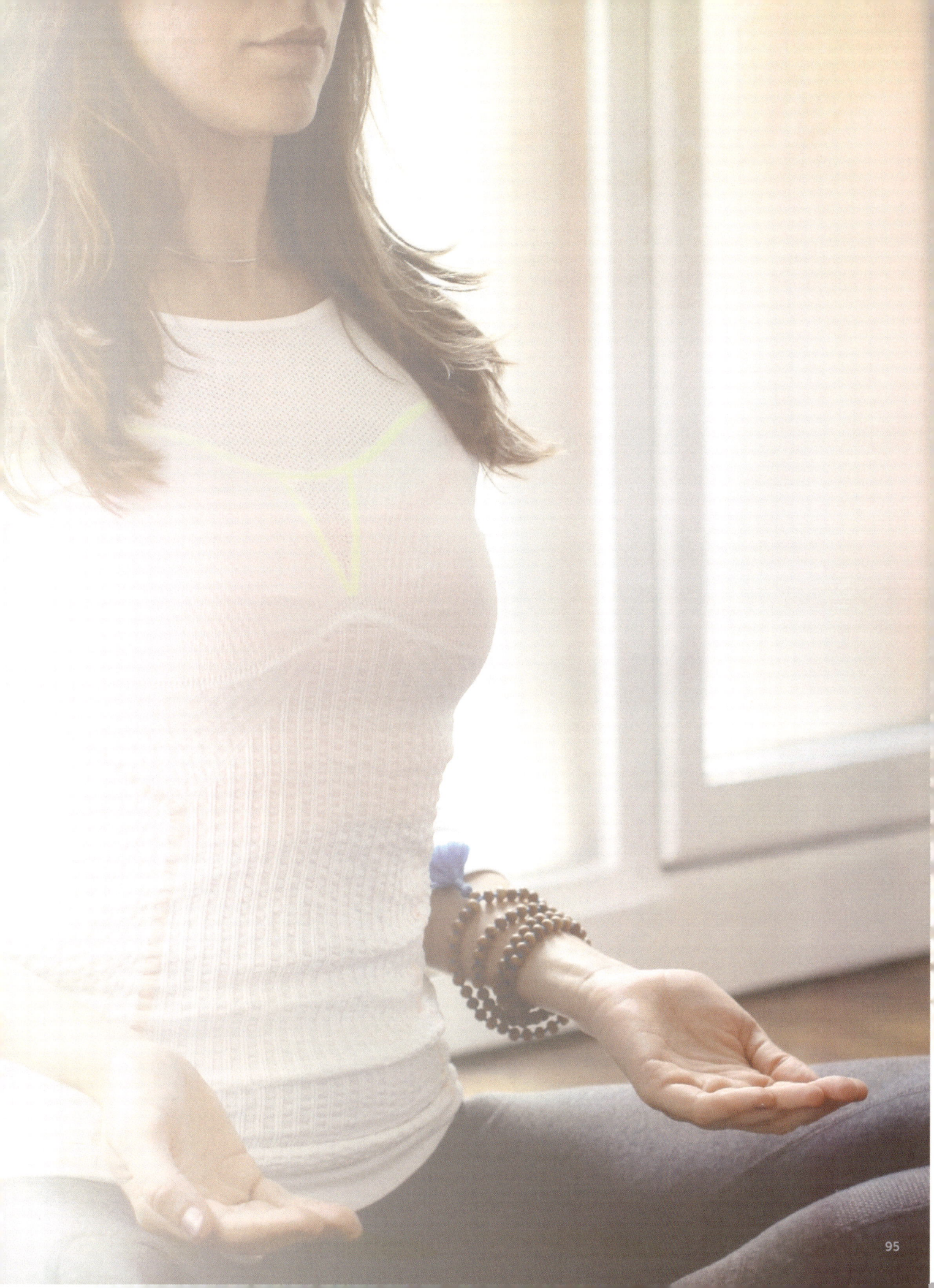

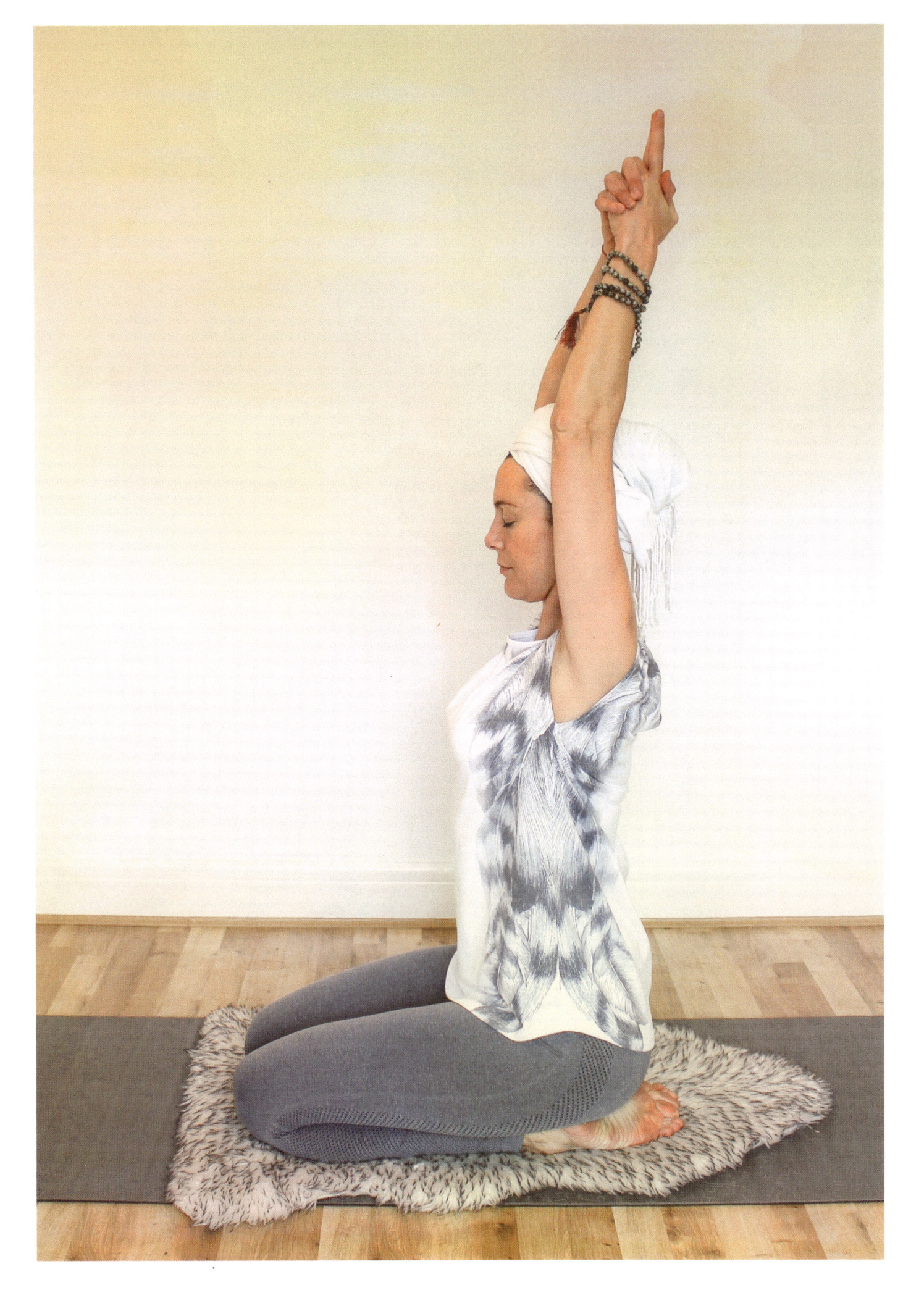

7

THE AURA

BAGGAGE OR ELEVATION

The magnetic field that surrounds your body can either trap you in patterns of reaction (your baggage) or bring awareness to protect and uplift in each moment with transparency.

#embodyyoursoulpurpose

@roisinallanakiernan

THE AURA
BAGGAGE OR ELEVATION

People tend to put a lot of emphasis on The Aura (the Seventh Body) – they want to see or feel them – but really what the Aura holds is your baggage. It's the magnetic field that surrounds your body and contained within that are all your pulsating rhythms, your patterns or trigger-like responses.

Have you ever met someone and disliked them for no apparent reason? Subconsciously there will have been an energetic interchange going on between the two of you. You'll have been triggered by something held in their aura, or vice versa. When you start to tune into your energetic reactions – when you give yourself space to feel the changes taking place in your body – then you can start to become more aware of these subconscious reactions and choose to act instead.

Every seven years your body goes through a complete new cycle. When you make positive changes to your patterns (thus changing part of your Aura) then you positively affect seven generations before and after you. Seven, therefore, is seen as a number of structure – it represents the structure of life in terms of karma. Seven is also the number of the upper astral plane, the place where spirits wait to enter a body holding the patterns necessary to process their karma. The law of karma is cause and effect, they're patterns that repeat themselves from the past into the future, through generations, over and over, until they're healed. Once healed, however, then our structure, or our Aura, is reshaped and our magnetic field – what we're putting out – changes.

Your Aura (magnetic field) can either trap you in patterns or you can feel into your triggers and choose to change.

When out of balance, your ego-mind will compensate and try to protect you (keep you trapped in your patterns) by projecting your inferiority or superiority complexes through The Aura. When in balance you believe in the truth of equality – you're able to stay with your energy and recognise that of another, without giving either the projective force to recreate patterns – you hold a clear, radiant magnetic field.

The Aura works as part of your defence system – alerting you to feelings that have previously caused you hurt. Unconscious patterns project out from all of us, until we take the time to become aware, understand and then hold them in the past.

Through the breath you can bring yourself into the present moment, taking every situation as a stand-alone occasion, rather than attaching your baggage onto it. By doing this, a transparency will develop – you'll be clear of the dramas that have held you in the past – and you can then offer a space of equality for the moment and person with whom you're engaging. As you develop this ability to breathe into each present moment then the patterns will fall away.

99

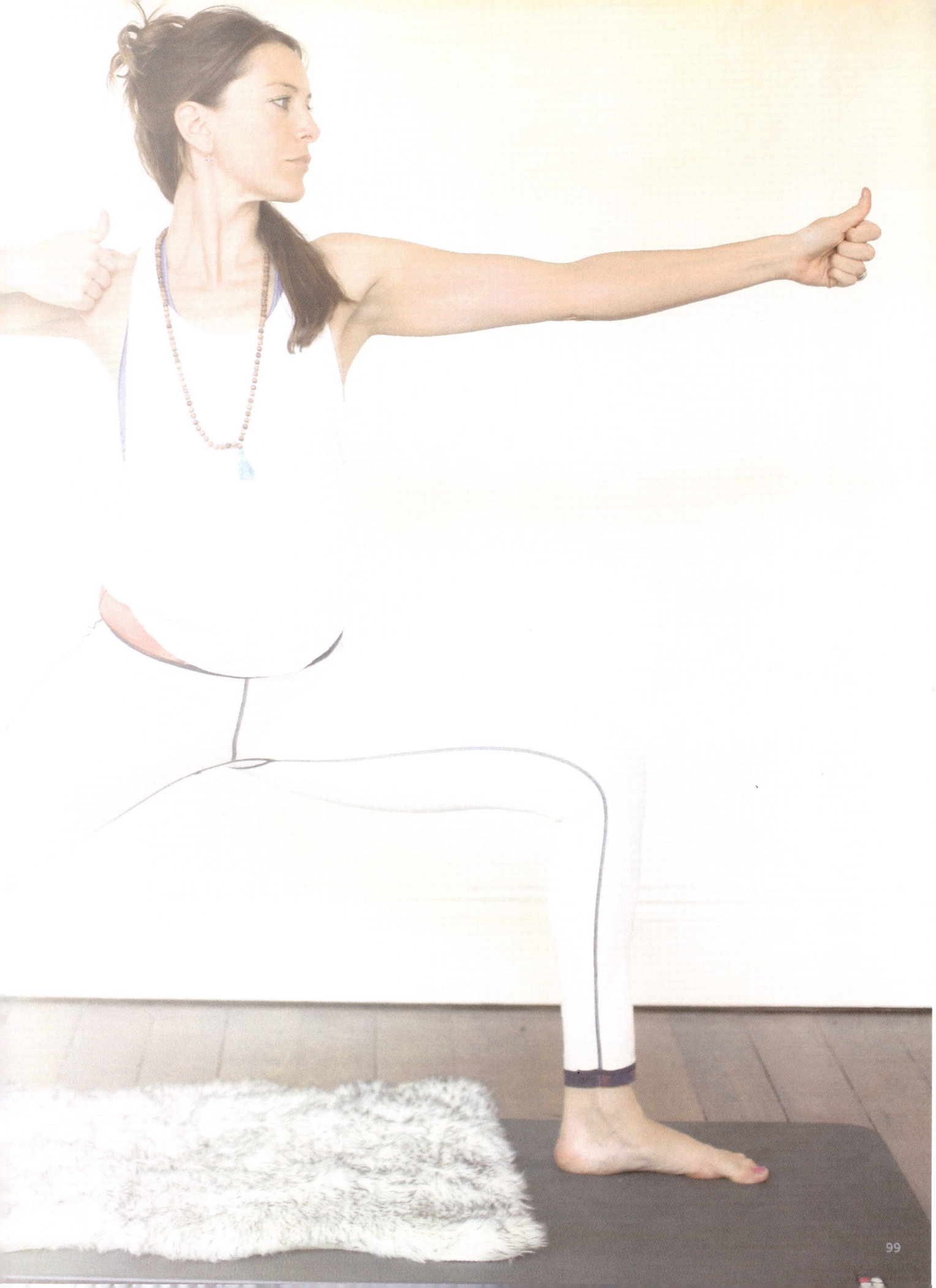

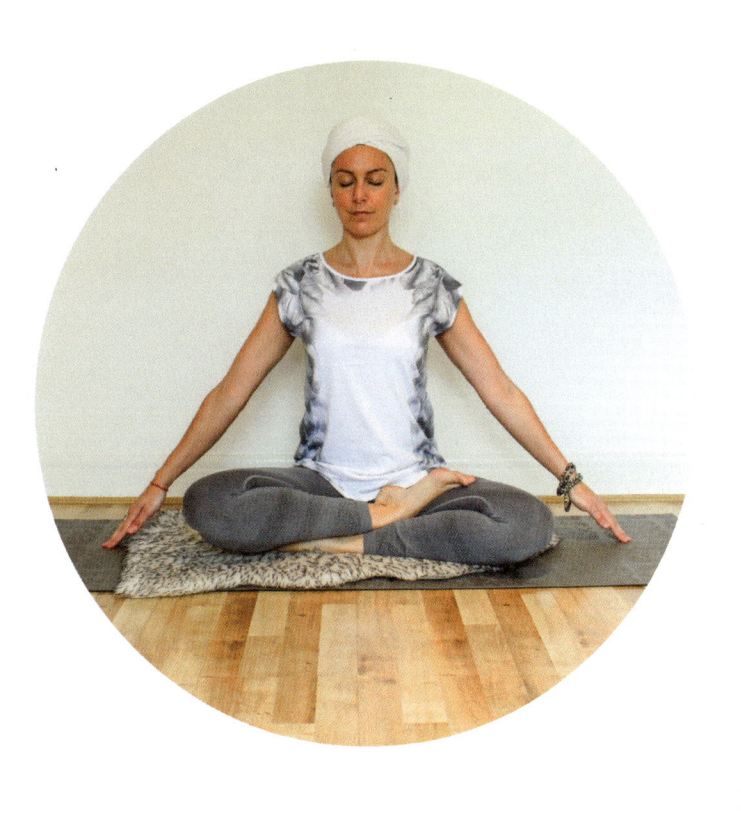

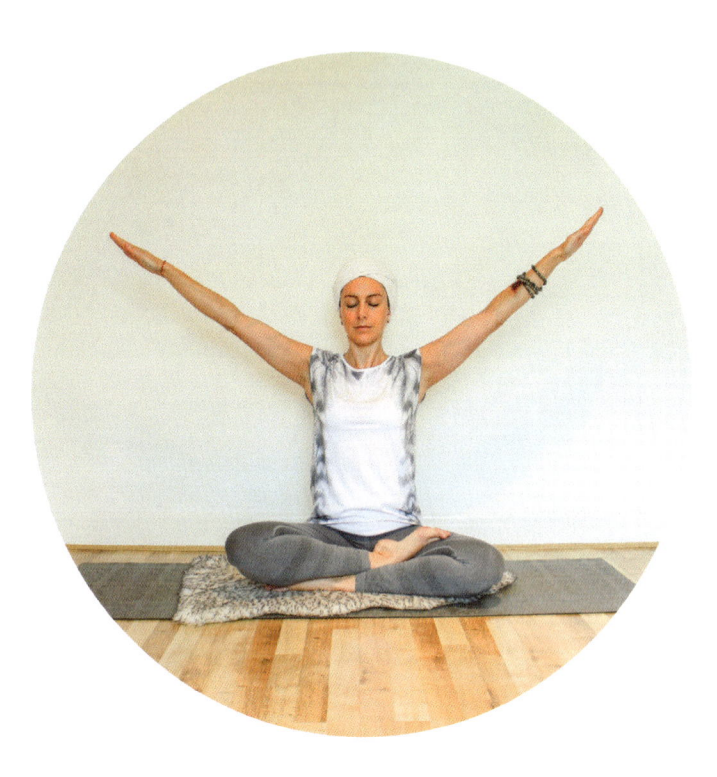

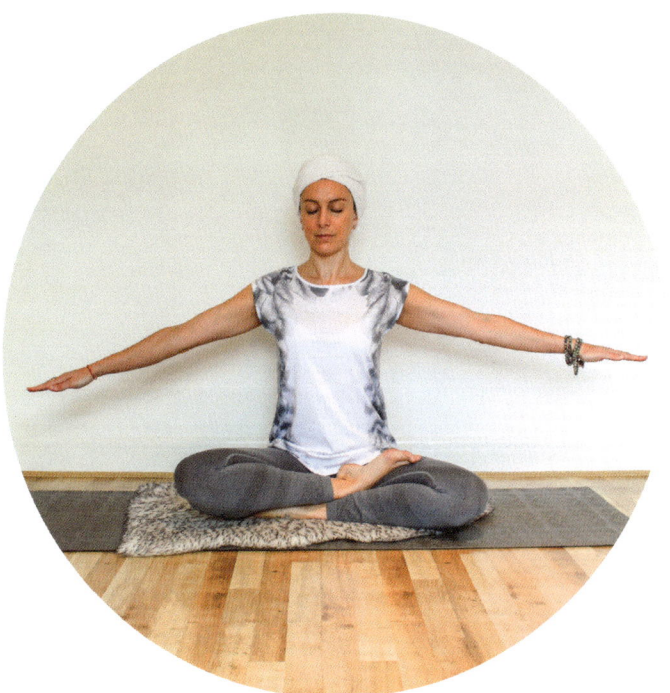

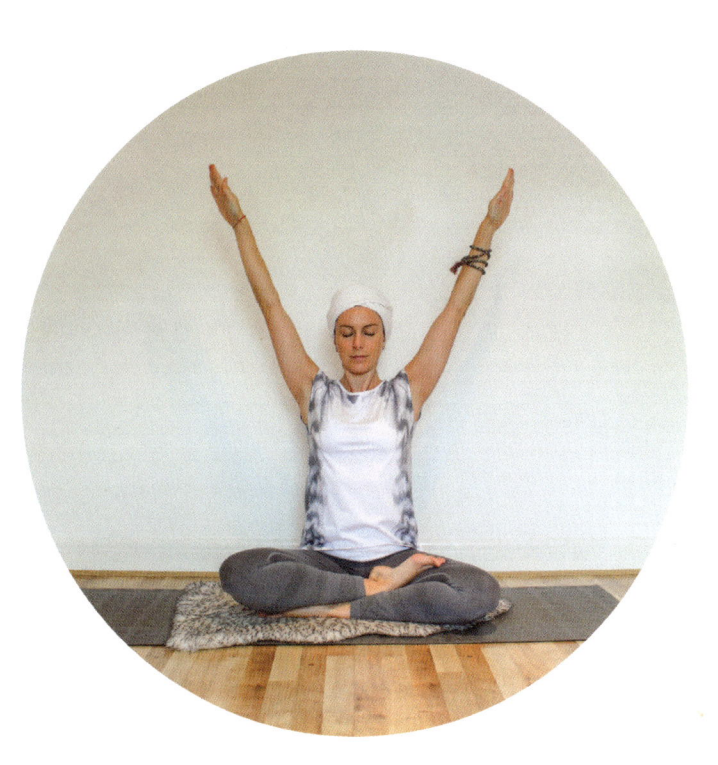

PRANAYAMA
AURA BUILDER

POSITION

Sitting with a tall spine, place your hands at your sides with straight elbows. You're going to inhale whilst raising your arms in four equal parts and movements. Then exhale and bring your arms down in one steady breath. Inhaling about 20 degrees for each part until the backs of your hands are almost touching above the head before you exhale slowly down.

The arms stay straight the whole time.

As you're moving, become aware of the space you occupy around your body – breathe into that space; reoccupy that space. Build your electromagnetic field to protect and project your truth; to move beyond your baggage.

DURATION

Minimum 3 Minutes

COMMENTS

This works to alleviate feelings of depression as it lifts you out of your baggage in The Aura – it expands you beyond. It also develops coordination, which develops the frontal brain, helping you to act in each moment, rather than following reactionary neural pathways (habitual behaviour).

#embodyyoursoulpurpose
@roisinallanakiernan

KRIYA

FOR S.A.D AND DEPRESSION

This Kriya will alleviate mild depression and Seasonal Affective Disorder (S.A.D). It also works to expand The Aura.

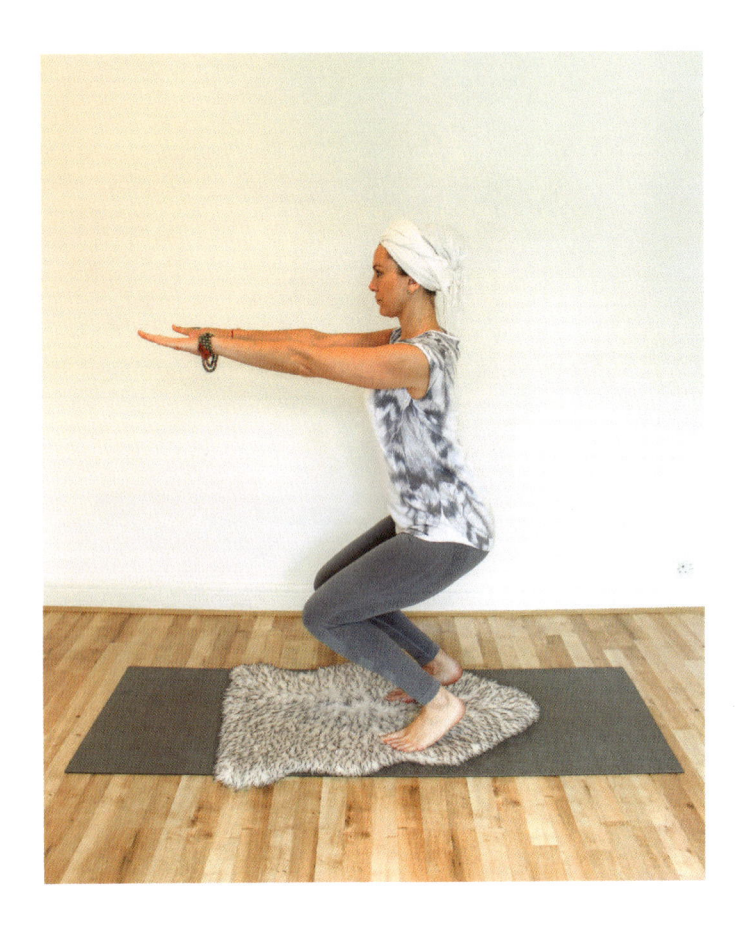

1. Squats on Tiptoes 2 Minutes

Instructions: Standing with your feet hip distance apart, bring the arms straight out from the shoulders, palms facing down and push up onto your tiptoes – that's your inhale position. Exhale (staying on the toes) into a squat – chest lifted, shoulders back and thighs parallel to the ground. Continue, inhaling up, exhaling down.

Benefits: This is great for your circulation, strengthens the knees and quads, and energises the sex nerve (inner thigh) and life nerve (sciatic).

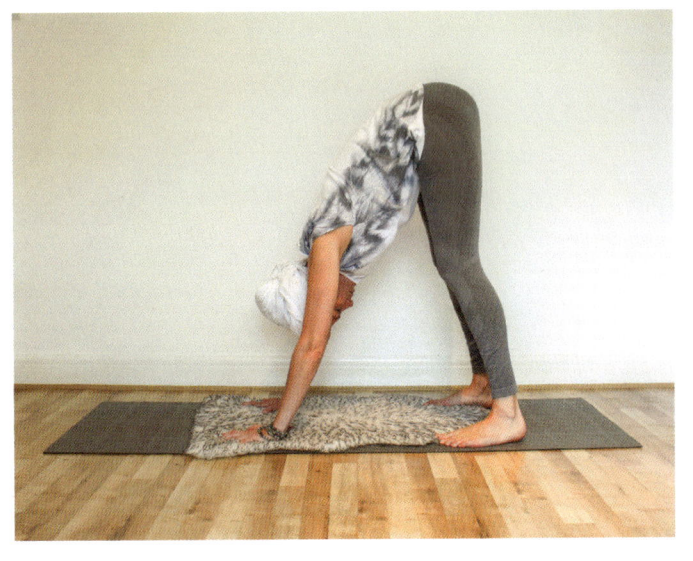

2. Elephant Walk 3 Minutes

Instructions: Remain standing up. Bend over and place the hands on the ground. Keeping the knees as straight as possible begin walking around the room on the hands and the feet. Let the breath regulate itself. Normal breath.

Benefits: This quickly eases any feelings of depression. It releases tension, stretches the whole body and strengthens the arms.

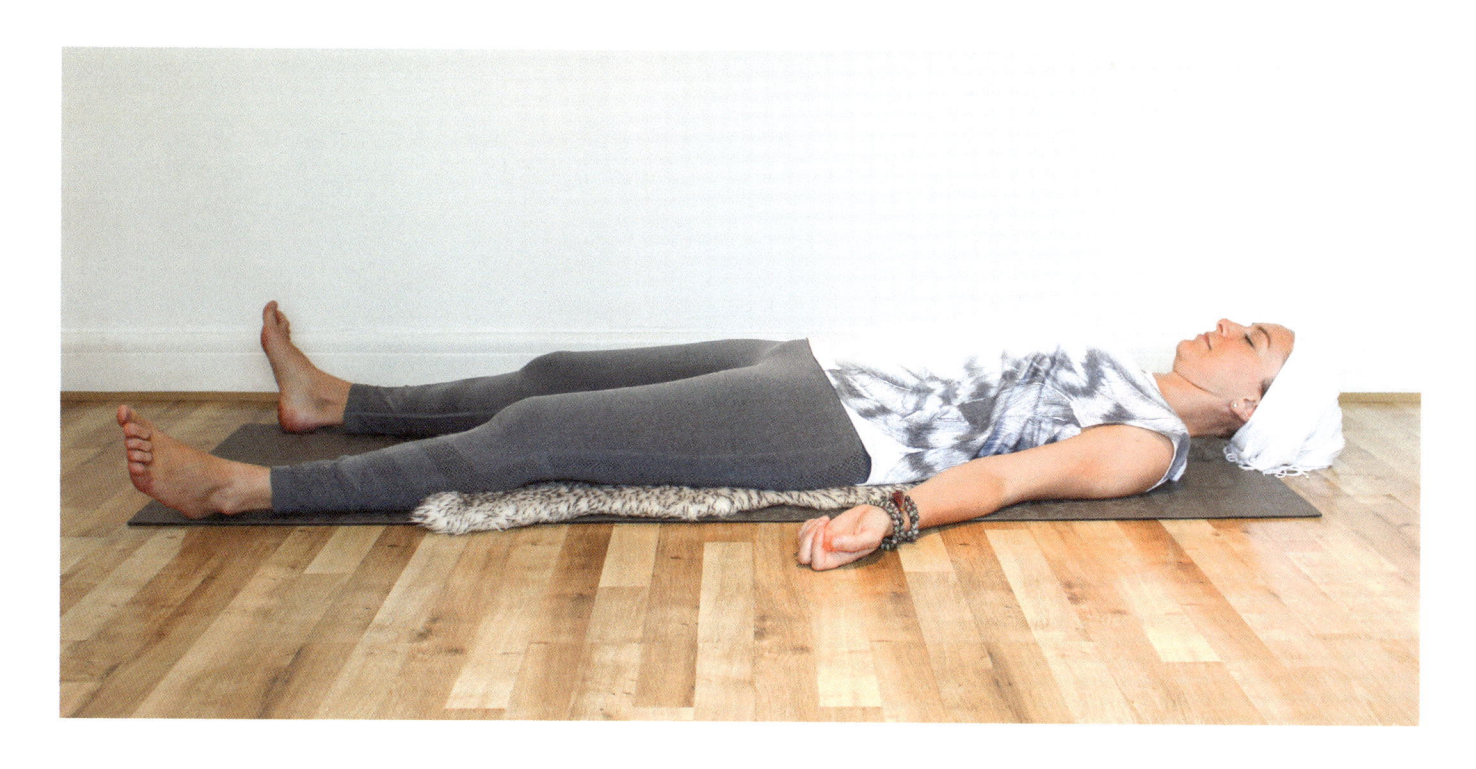

3. Relax in Corpse Pose (Shavasana) 2 Minutes

Instructions: Lie on your back, legs uncrossed and hands out by your sides, palms up. Relax.

Meditation: With every inhalation feel more and more love radiating from your heart centre and flowing through your system.

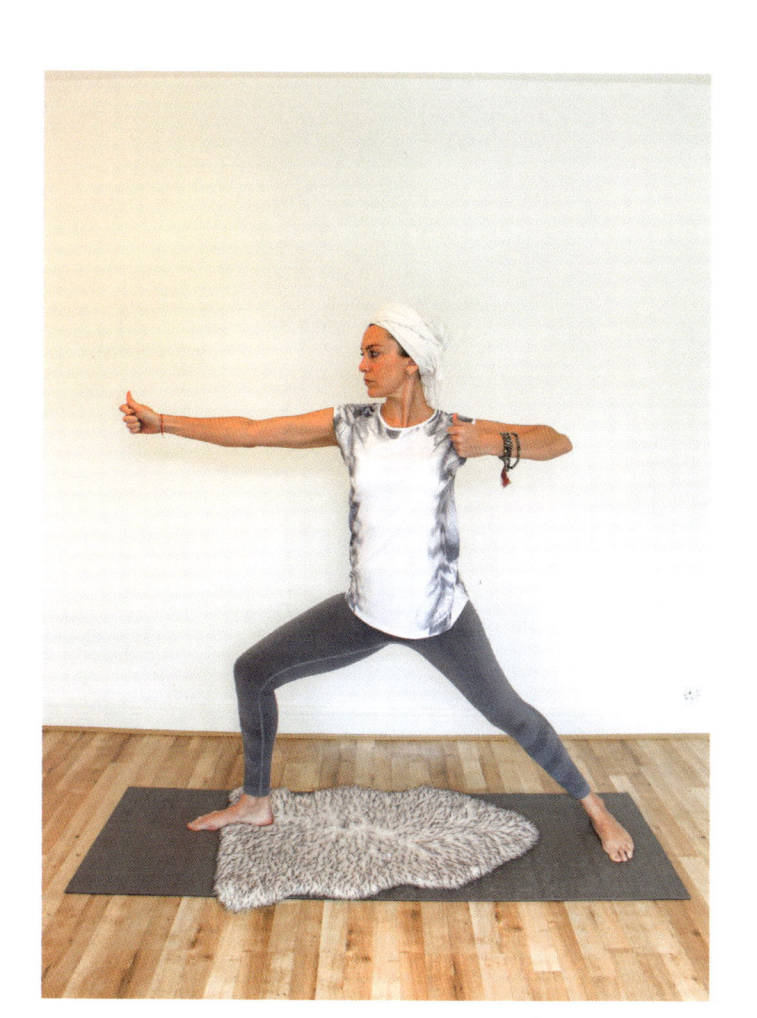

4. Archer Pose (Warrior 2) – Both Sides
2 Minutes on Each Side

Instructions: Standing at the back of your mat, take a long step forward with your left leg. Turn the back foot out to bring it flat – the leg stays straight. Bend your front knee, making sure it comes directly above your ankle. Then, with hands in fists and thumbs up, imagine you're pulling a bow and arrow from a bag on your back. Hold the bow out with your left hand – arm held parallel to the ground – and from that bow pull your arrow back to your right shoulder with your right hand. The right elbow remains up in line with the shoulder, your chest opens and head turns so your eyes can focus on the thumb of the left hand. Hold this position and breathe long and slow. Then change sides.

Benefits: This pose builds confidence and courage. It also works to stretch and strengthen the whole body. It's a Warrior pose, so your whole body should be engaged and ready.

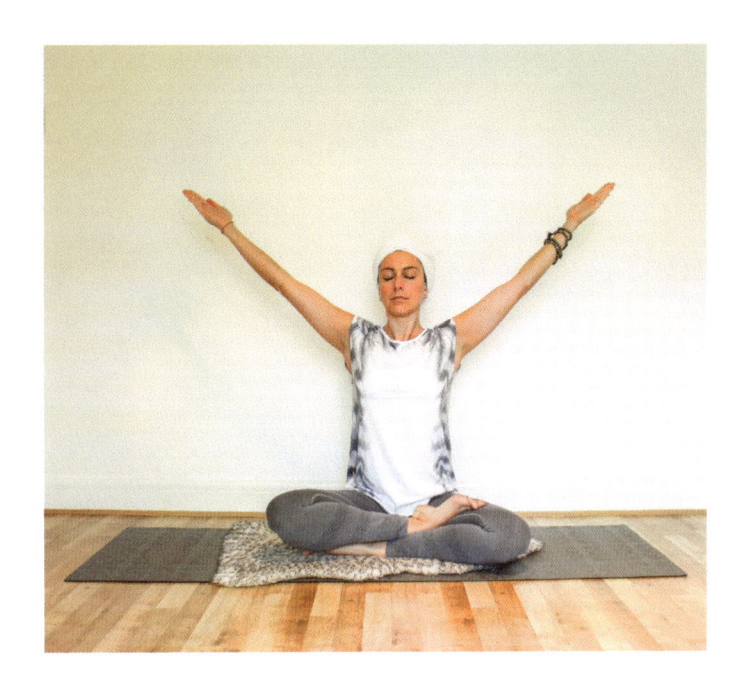

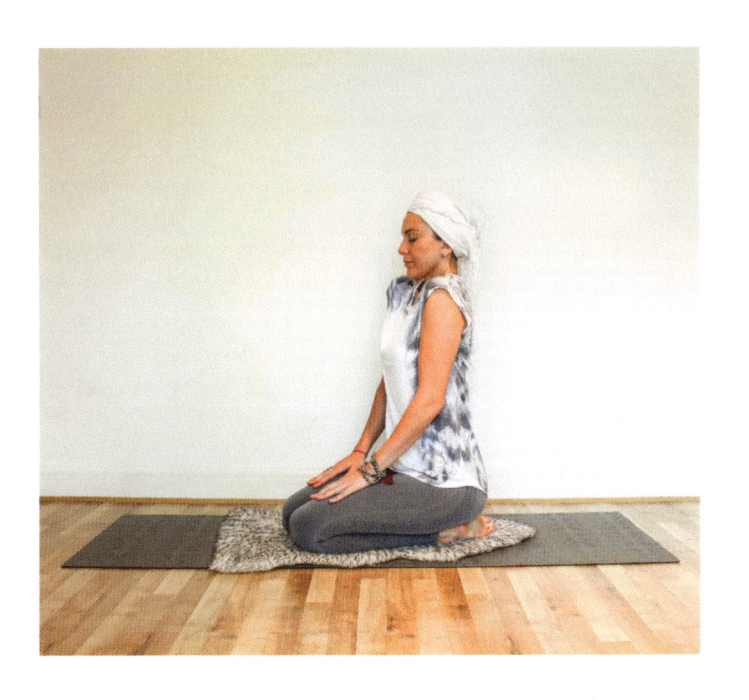

5. Aura Builder   1 Minute

Instructions: Seated with a tall spine, bring your arms out to the sides and raise them up to a sixty-degree angle. The elbows are straight, palms flat and facing towards each other overhead. Bring your attention to the space up between the palms and concentrate on building the energy and light between them, using Breath of Fire (rapid breathing in and out of the nose, using your navel to pump the breath) to push your energy (or will power) up to the space between the hands.

Benefits: This expands and strengthens the energy field around the body.

6. Aura Extender   1 Minute

Instructions: Remain sitting tall but bring your arms down in line with the shoulders, elbows stay straight but bend the wrists so your hands push out, fingers pointing up towards the sky. Hold this position with Breath of Fire.

Benefits: This also works to expand and strengthen your energy field.

7. Shoulder Rolls   1 Minute

Instructions: Seated with your hands on the knees, roll your shoulders together in big, slow circles. The breath will find its own flow.

Benefits: This eases off any tension in the shoulders and opens the chest, heart and throat.

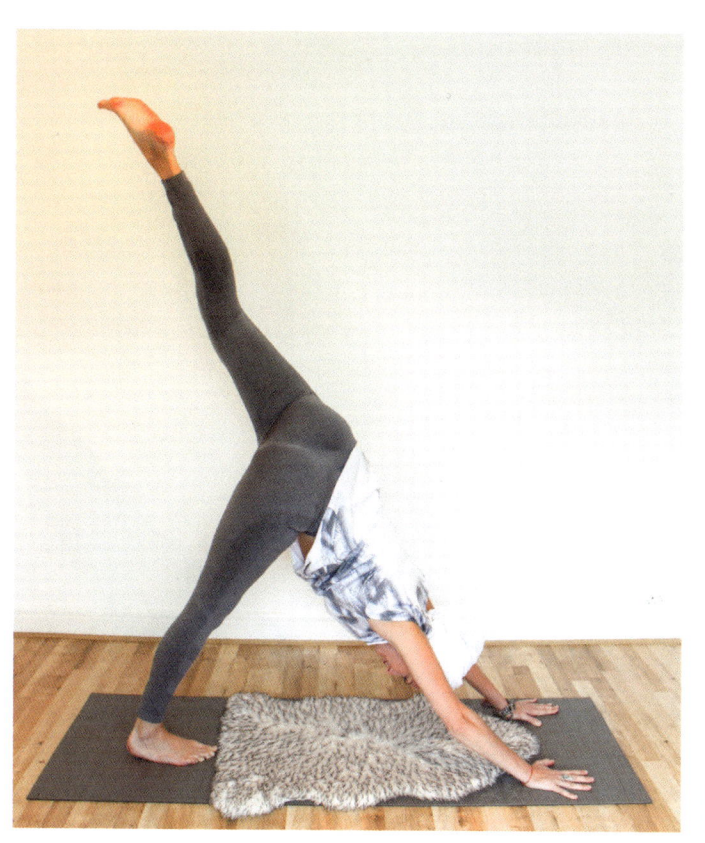

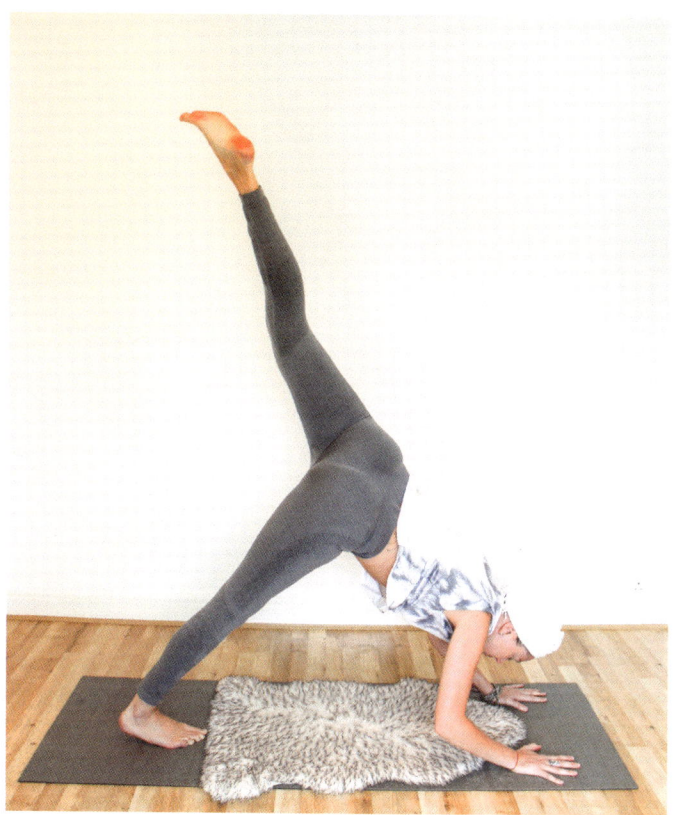

8. Triangle Pose Push Ups   6-10 Push Ups on Each Side

Instructions: From your hands and knees, push up into Triangle Pose (Down Dog). Spread your fingers and push back with the hands, allow the chest to drop and the hips to rise. You might like to bend one knee after the other a while to stretch the hamstrings if they feel tight. Then, lifting the left leg as high and as straight as possible, do push-ups in this position – inhaling in the original position and exhaling as you bend the elbows and ease your position down as far as you can, before inhaling up again and continuing. Then change sides.

Benefits: This builds your whole body aura and strengthens your upper body strength.

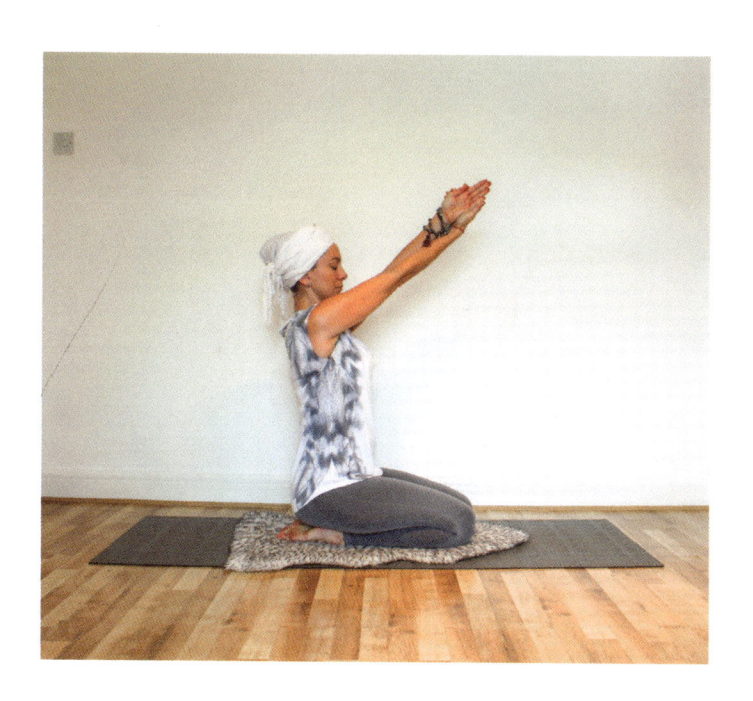

9. Front Arm Pumps   90 Seconds

Instructions: Sit on the knees and heels or simply with a straight spine if this seated position isn't possible. Then, bring your left arm out in front of you, with the palm facing to your right – as if you're about to shake hands. Then, reach the right arm under the left, grabbing the back of the left hand. Keep your arms straight and in this hand position whilst continuously inhaling them up to sixty degrees and exhaling them down.

Benefits: This strengthens the upper body, releases any tension in the shoulders and works to 'cut through' any baggage in The Aura.

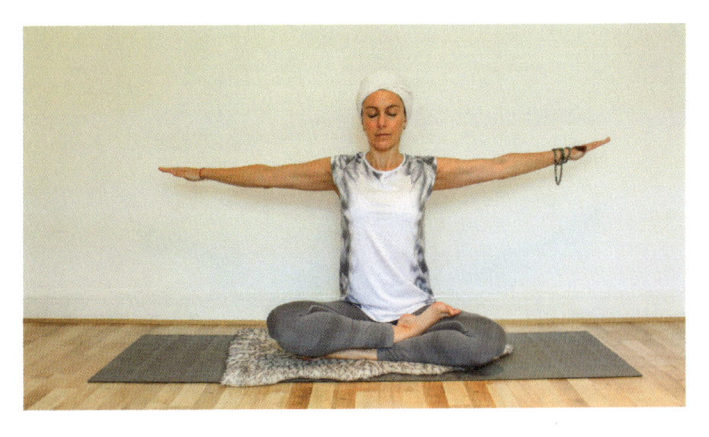

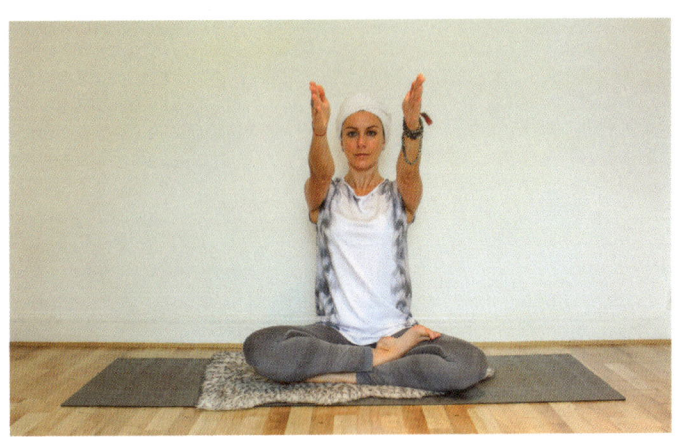

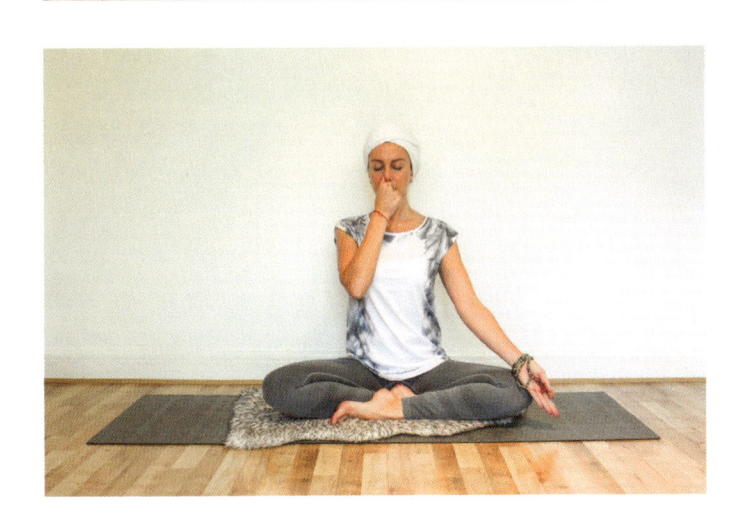

10. Arm Swings 2 Minutes

Instructions: Sitting with a straight spine and eyes closed, inhale and swing the arms back – your palms are facing the ground – then exhale and bring the hands in front of the face, palms facing each other. When your palms are in front of the face, about two inches apart, open your eyes and look in between them. Then, again, close the eyes and swing the arms back before continuing.

Benefits: This works to expand the front and sides of The Aura and assists your ability to see auras. It also loosens the shoulders and opens up the lungs.

11. Silent Resting Meditation 30 Seconds

Instructions: Sit quietly, breathing long and deep and feel into the space around your body – try to sense your electromagnetic field (your aura); picturing it as light and expanded energy around your physical body.

Benefits: This helps to consolidate and brings greater awareness to The Aura.

12. Balanced Breath Meditation

2 Minutes

Instructions: Seated with a tall spine, use your right hand to close the right nostril and inhale through the left. Then, using the same hand, block off your left nostril and exhale right. Inhale right, exhale left; inhale left, exhale right; and so on.
Use long, slow, deep breathing.

Benefits: This revitalises the nervous system, balances the hemispheres of the brain and generally calms you.

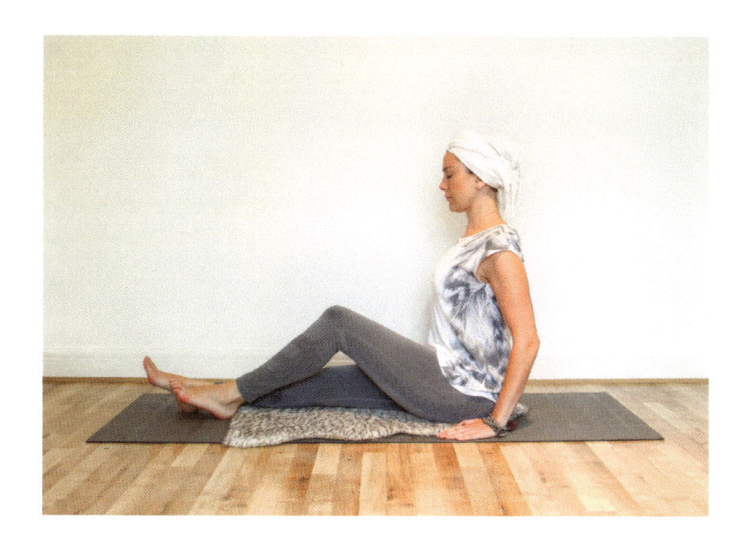

13. Leg Shake   30 Seconds

Instructions: Seated, stretch your legs out in front of you and shake them.

Benefits: This is good for the hips and adjusts the sacrum area (lower back).

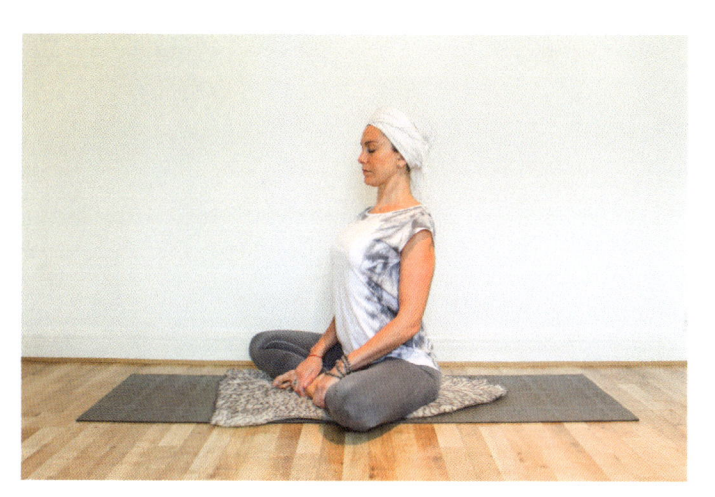

14. Spinal Flex   3 Minutes

Instructions: Sitting with a tall spine and, keeping your head in line with the base of your spine, inhale through the nose as you arch the torso forward – opening the chest and drawing the shoulders back, then exhale through the nose and round the back.

Benefits: This works to bring strength and flexibility to the lower back. After 3 minutes, the brain wave patterns change, making you more calm.

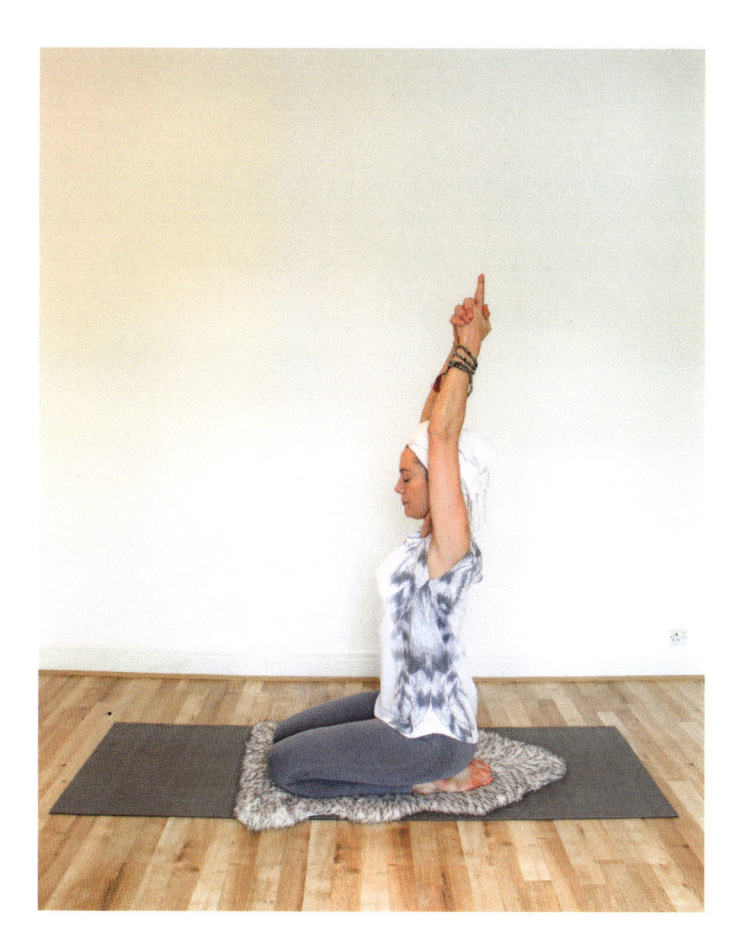

15. Sat Kriya   3 Minutes

Instructions: Sitting in the knees, on the heels, or with a straight spine, as you can. Bring your arms up over head, interlace the fingers except the index fingers, which point straight up. Ladies, cross your left thumb over right. Gents, right over left. Eyes are closed.

In this position, you're going to chant 'Sat Nam' (True Name). Chant Sat as you pull the navel in (using your will power there to help you step up to your truth). Then, as the energy rises to the Third Eye (in and up between the brows), gently, chant Nam.
The breath will find its own way.

Benefits: This meditation is fundamental to the practise of Kundalini Yoga, because it works to directly raise the Kundalini energy – your dormant creative potential. The rhythmic contraction and relaxation of the navel produces waves of energy that circulate, energise and heal the body.

MEDITATION

THE DIVINE SHIELD MEDITATION FOR PROTECTION AND POSITIVITY

POSITION

Sitting with a straight spine, raise your right knee, leaving your right foot flat on the floor, toes pointing forward. You left leg is bent at the knee, with the sole of the foot against the inside of the right foot.

Your left hand rests on the floor beside you, supporting you as your right hand is drawn up beside the face. Use your right hand to 'cup' the ear – as if to amplify a sound you want to hear. The face remains looking forward with eyes closed.

In this position, inhale deeply and chant 'Maaa' with long, full, smooth sounds. In a group setting, each person inhales when they need so a continuous sound is created.

Chant at a comfortably high pitch and listen to the sound - let it vibrate through your whole body.

MANTRA

Maaa

DURATION

11 – 31 minutes on each side

Start slowly – learn to hold the concentration of the sound – and build to 62 minutes on each side.

TO END

Inhale and stretch your hands up and back as far as possible. Hold for 10-15 seconds then exhale. Repeat 3 times. And relax.

COMMENTS

Maa is the same sound a baby uses to call for its mother. In this meditation, your soul is the child and the Universe your Mother. Call on the Divine Mother to support and protect you. Practised daily, this meditation will bring positivity and fearlessness. It will remove any feelings of separation and assist you in pursuing your goals.

When our Aura is weak, we can feel depressed and isolated; we're fearful and easily drawn down by other's emotions. This meditation expands The Aura and activates the power of the Heart Centre, by connecting it with the universal field through mantra. In this way, you align with universal love, allowing life to flow as it comes and goes, without being pulled down by the storms that pass through.

#embodyyoursoulpurpose

@roisinallanakiernan

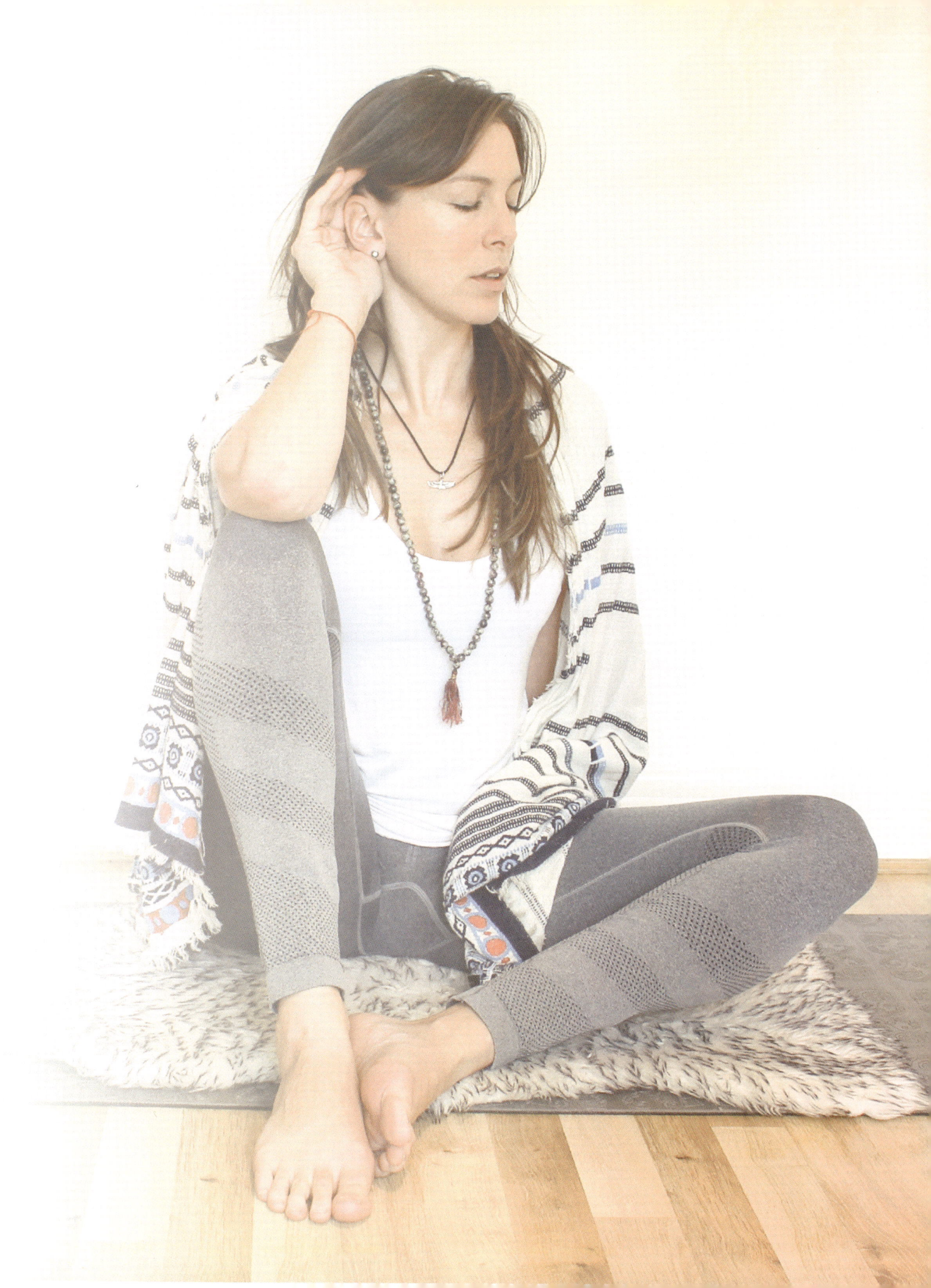

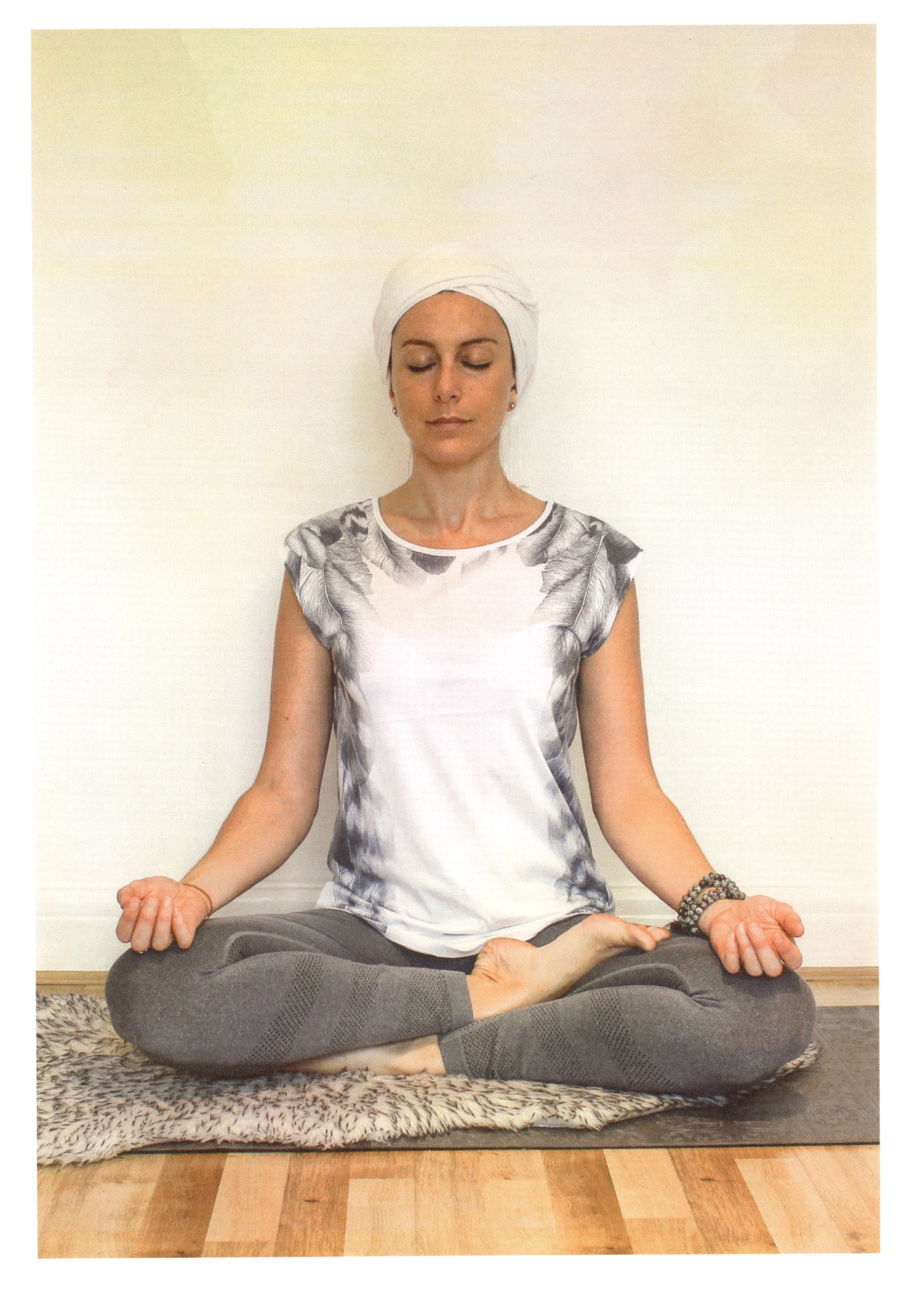

8

THE PRANIC BODY

THE INFINITE BREATH

Prana is the life force energy we take in through the breath, which flows in and out like the tide, coming and going, moment to moment. We can either flow with it or create resistance through fear and control, leading to illness.

#embodyyoursoulpurpose

@roisinallanakiernan

THE PRANIC BODY
THE INFINITE BREATH

Eight is the number of the Infinite – two circles flowing in and out of each other in continuous, connected movement. You can choose this constant, abundant flow of life, moment to moment, inhale to exhale, breath by breath, from the finite into infinity and back. Or you can create resistance through fear and control, which ultimately leads to illness.

The eighth body is the Pranic Body – Prana being the energy that you get from the breath as you inhale and exhale, like the tide washing in and drawing back, like the light and dark of day and night. Indeed, the number eight is symbolic of this push and pull, the Infinite movement of your soul and self through lifetimes, through the breath, through the Pranic Body.

You can learn to flow with life through the Pranic Body but, naturally, you'll also hit obstacles, build barriers and become stagnant at times. Finding a way for life to flow is key to a healthy life. Many illnesses are started through resistance to this flow, whereas healing can occur when you allow yourself to feel and move through the thoughts and feelings or causes of your illness – a death process in order to be reborn, just like the continuous cycle or flow of night and day.

A strong Pranic Body will give you a strong sense of self - will help you feel grounded, secure in yourself and see everyone as equal. You will feel connected with the Infinite nature of life – able to let go, trust and flow.

A weak Pranic Body will create a weak self-identity that tries to contain this life force energy (Prana) by demanding authority. An obsession with cleanliness would show a need to hold on or contain such Prana. On the flip-side, too much Prana can also lead to a day dreamy reality - a life with your head in the clouds.

If you're nervous or anxious (uncertain in your sense of self) then your breath can become shallow and restricted. Asthma can be a sign of such anxiety, often caused through a bad experience with the abuse of power or authority. Too much air and you can become ungrounded.

In order to balance your eighth, Pranic Body, you must live in the moment, bringing your dreams down to Earth and working with each situation as it comes, not forgetting your dreams but anchoring them in reality. Abundance cannot be contained, all must come and go and flow within each moment.

Your breath is key to this flow, just as the flow of your breath is key to recognising the flow of your life.

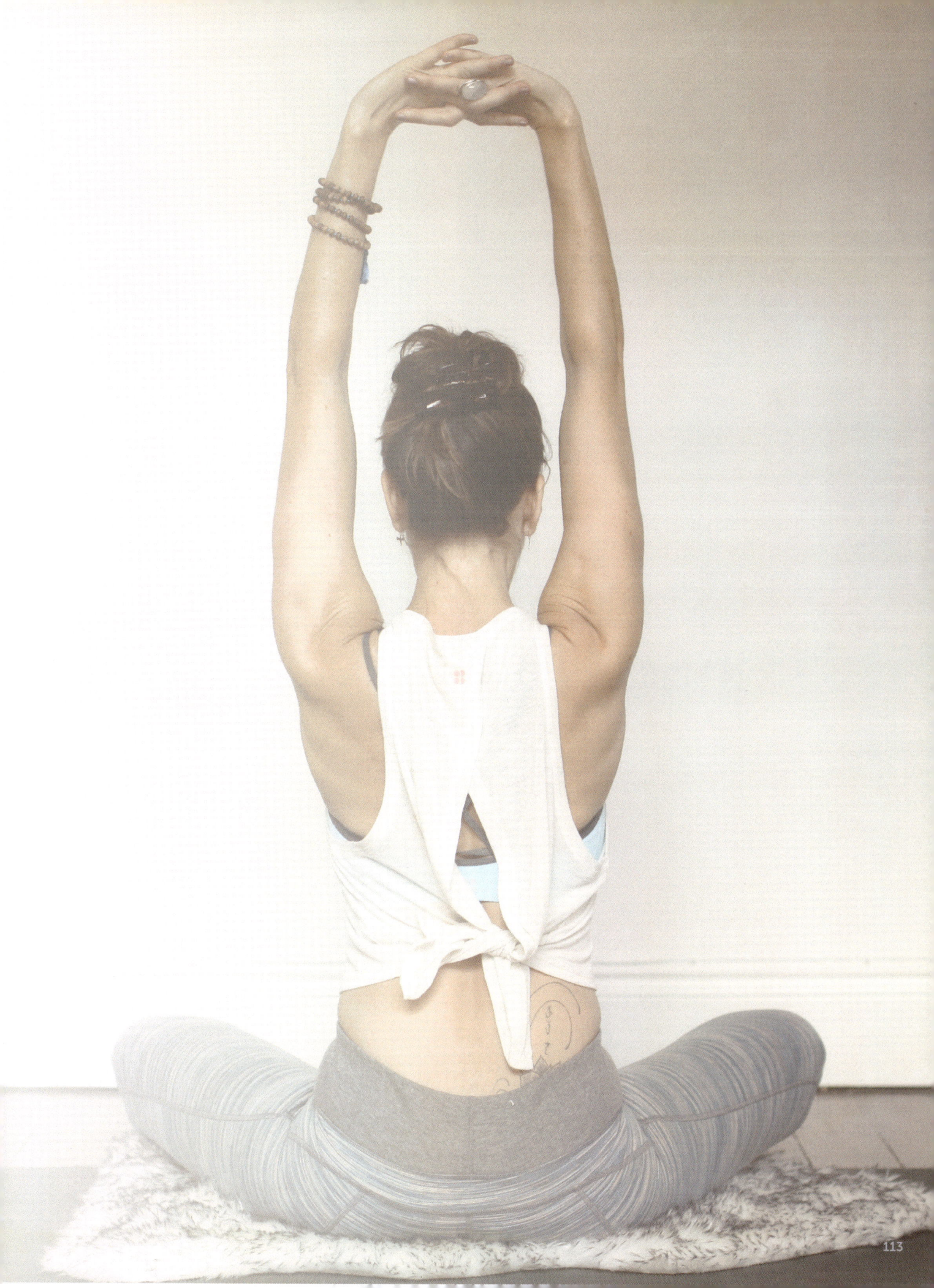

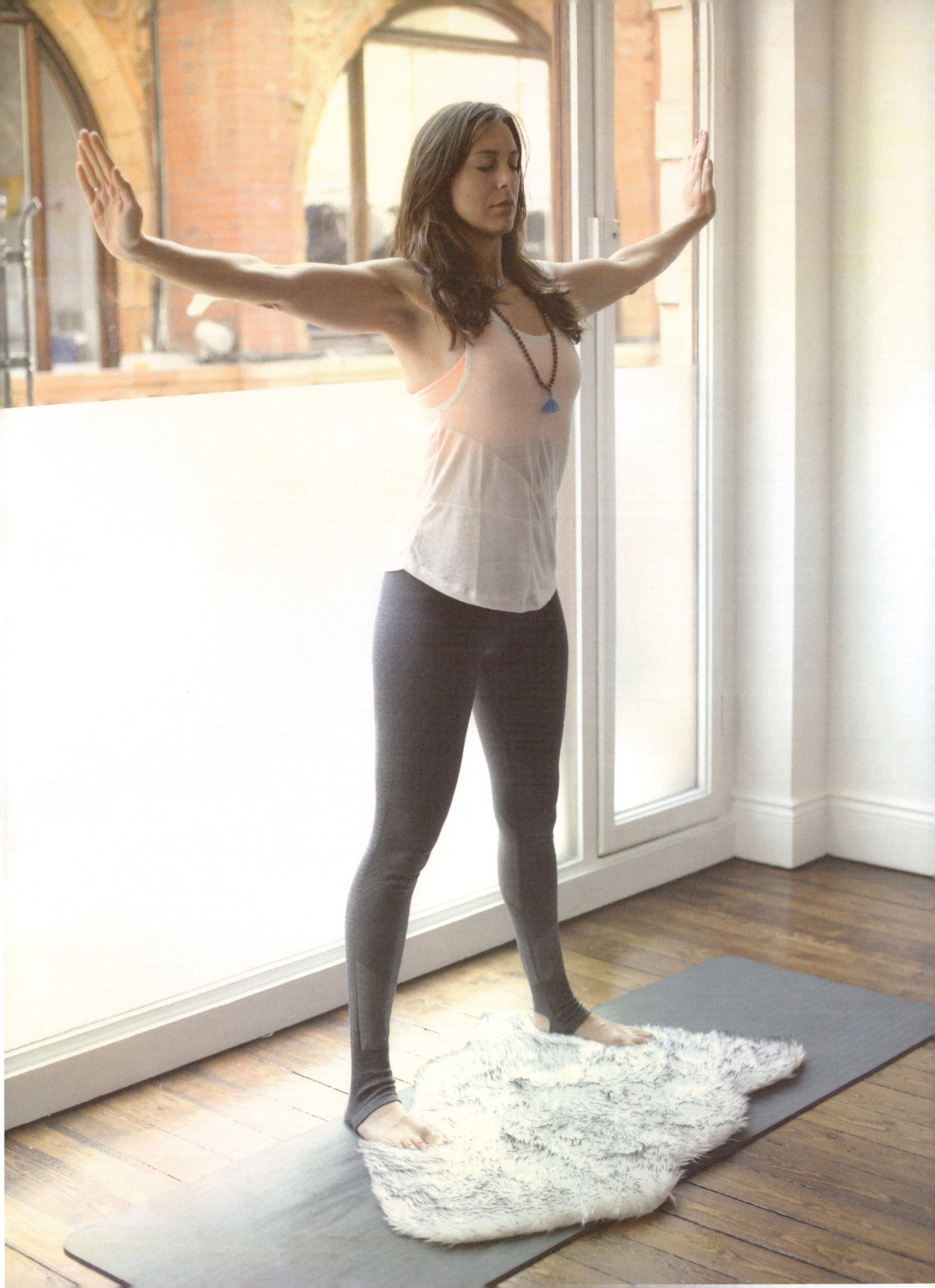

PRANAYAMA
BREATH OF FIRE EXPANSION

POSITION

Standing with your feet wide, bring your arms out straight from the shoulders and bend your wrists so your hands face out to the sides, fingers pointing up. Close the eyes and use a powerful Breath of Fire (rapidly breathing in and out of the nose, using your navel as a pump).

DURATION

3 Minutes

COMMENTS

This will expand your sense of self beyond the physical body into your energetic field.

NB: I have adapted this breathing exercise from Yogi Bhajan's teachings; he never taught Breath of Fire in this way.

#embodyyoursoulpurpose

@roisinallanakiernan

KRIYA

PREPARATORY EXERCISES FOR LUNGS, MAGNETIC FIELD AND DEEP MEDITATION

The first few exercises in this kriya work to purify the blood and expand the lung capacity. Then the circulatory system is stimulated, helping to release secretions from the thyroid and parathyroid glands. All work to enlarge the magnetic field and prepare you for deep meditation.

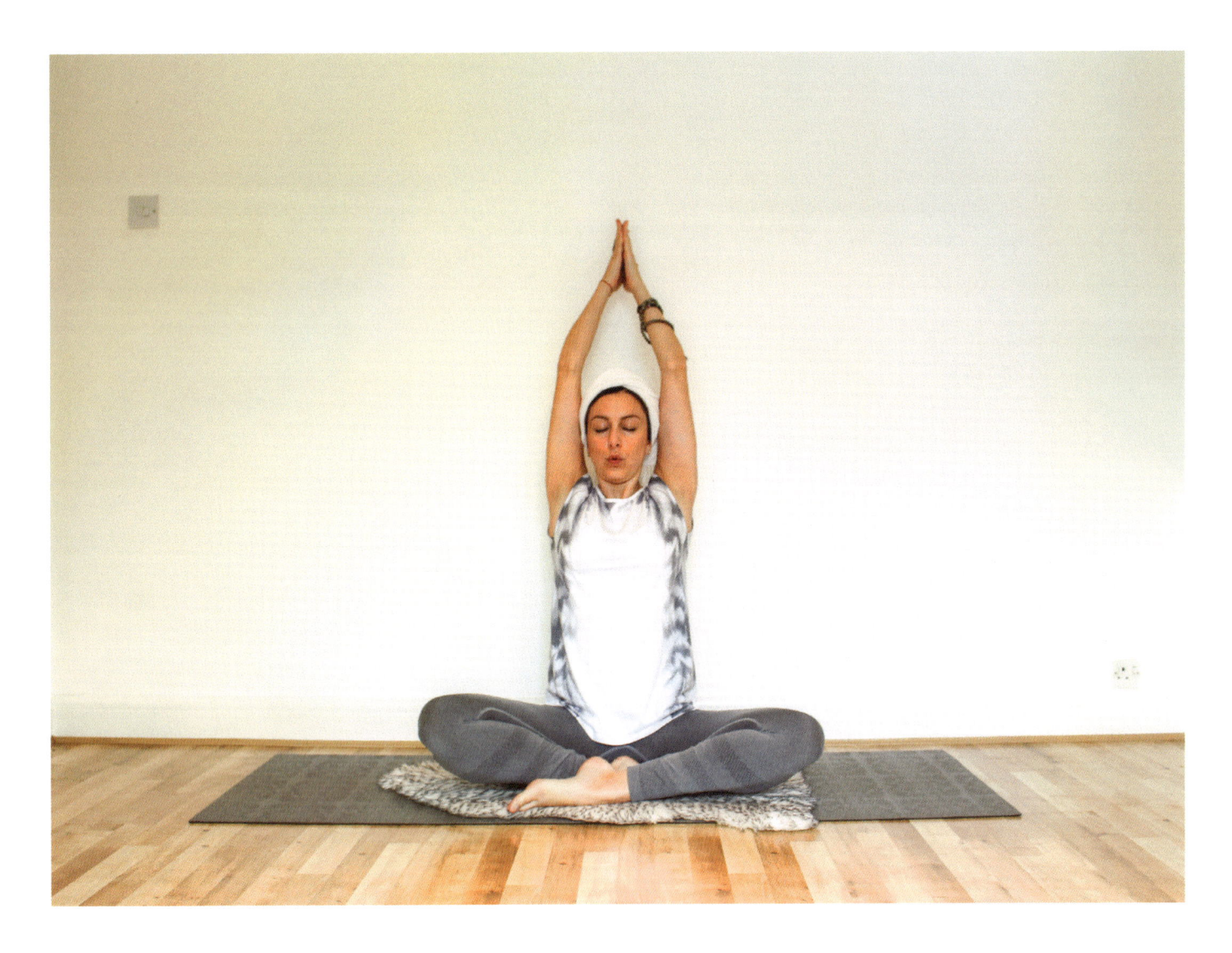

1. Whistle Breath   5 Minutes

Instructions: Sit with a tall spine and bring your arms straight up in prayer above the head. Lean back as far as you comfortably can and breathe in and out through puckered lips. To end, relax for 30 seconds.

Benefits: This stimulates the Vagus Nerve, which is the longest cranial nerve, running from the brain stem, down through the organs in the neck, chest and abdomen. It sends messages to everything from the neck down and can weaken through stress.

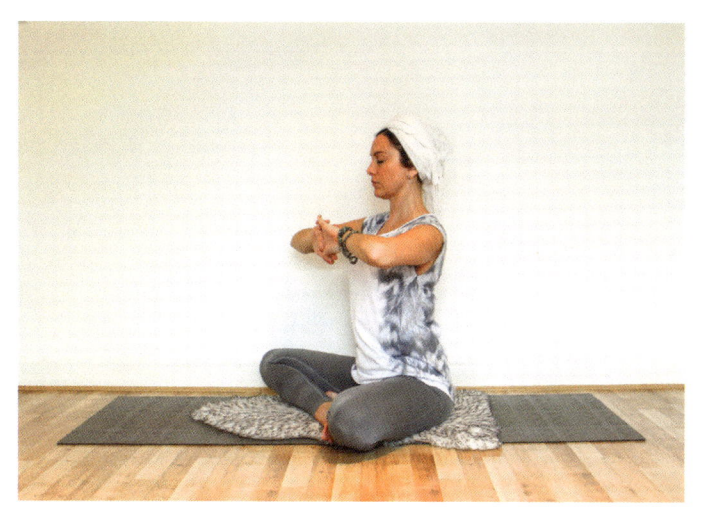

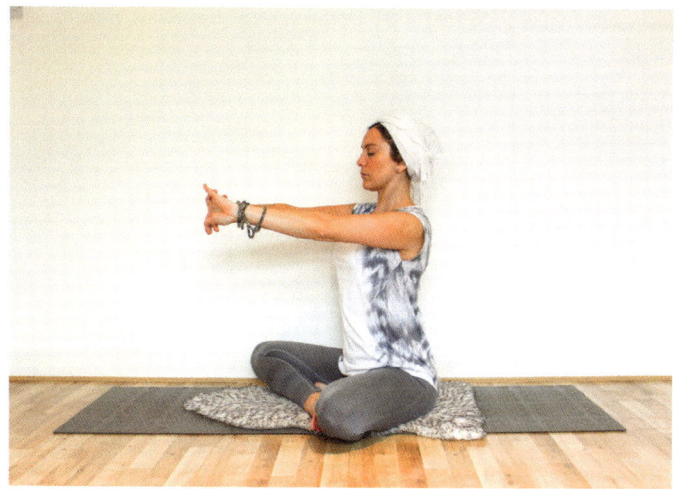

2. Arm Stretch 2-3 Minutes

Instructions: Sitting tall, interlace your fingers with the thumb tips touching and turn the hands so the palms face out from the heart space. Inhale as you straighten out the arms from the heart (keeping fingers interlaced) and exhale return to the original position. Continue rapidly – inhaling out, exhaling in.

To End: Inhale and hold the breath with the arms extended then, keeping the position, exhale and move straight into the next exercise.

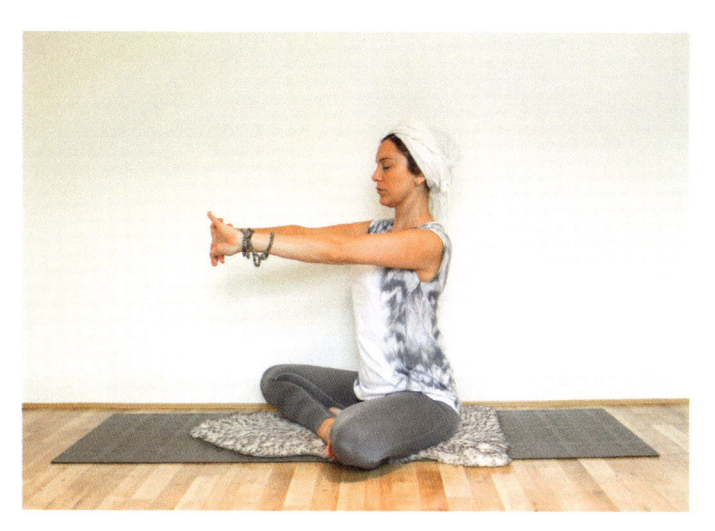

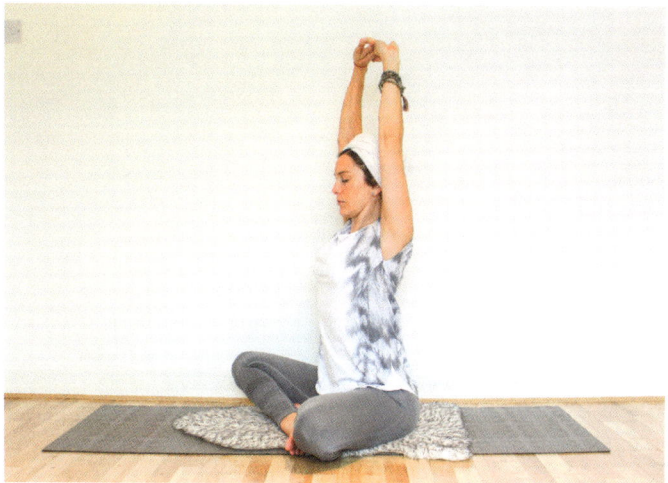

3. Arm Pumps 2-3 Minutes

Instructions: With the arms extended from the last exercise, inhale, hold the breath, and pump the arms up and down over the head. Then, when you need to, exhale the hands back to the chest – to the starting position from the last exercise.

To End: Inhale with the arms extended and hold briefly for 10-15 seconds.

Benefits: These arm exercises work to open up the shoulders, chest and heart and develop lung capacity.

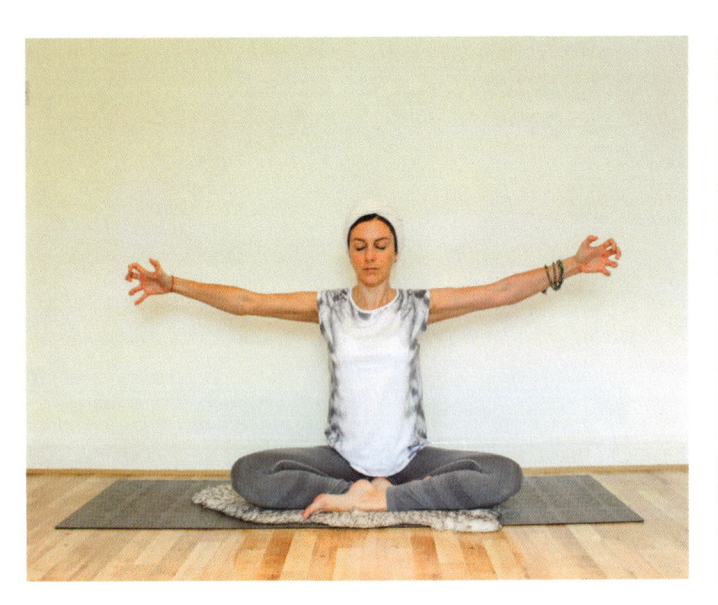

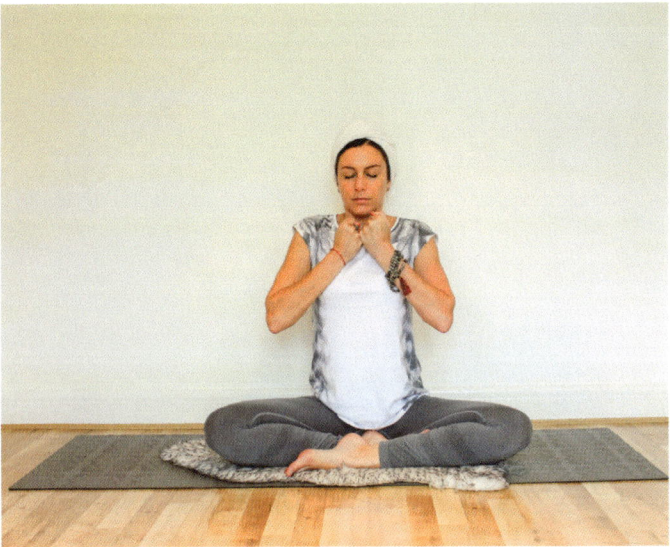

4. Arm Grabs 3 Minutes

Instructions: Immediately extend the arms straight out to the sides with the palms facing forward. As you inhale, start clenching the fists and, holding the breath, draw those clenched fists in towards the chest. As you draw them in, imagine they're carrying a heavy load – your baggage. When you reach the heart, release the breath and the hands explosively back to the start position.

Continue, bringing all your concentration to this great weight - your face should show the pain and determination involved in the task.

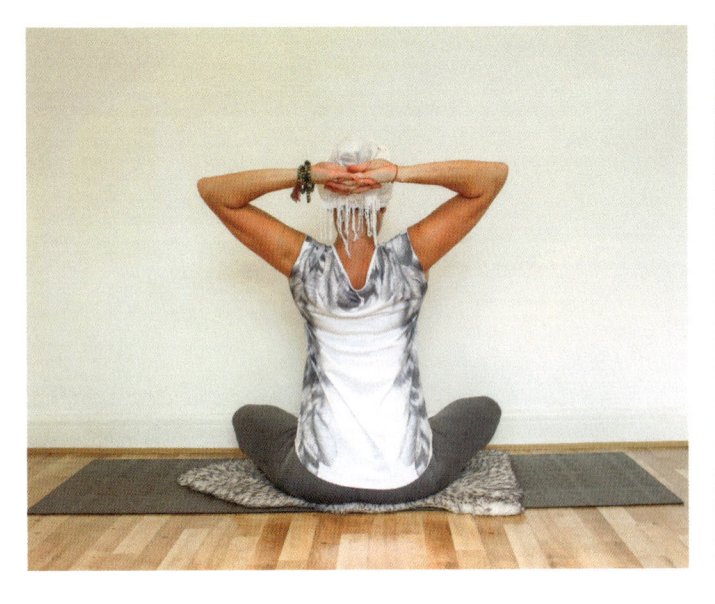

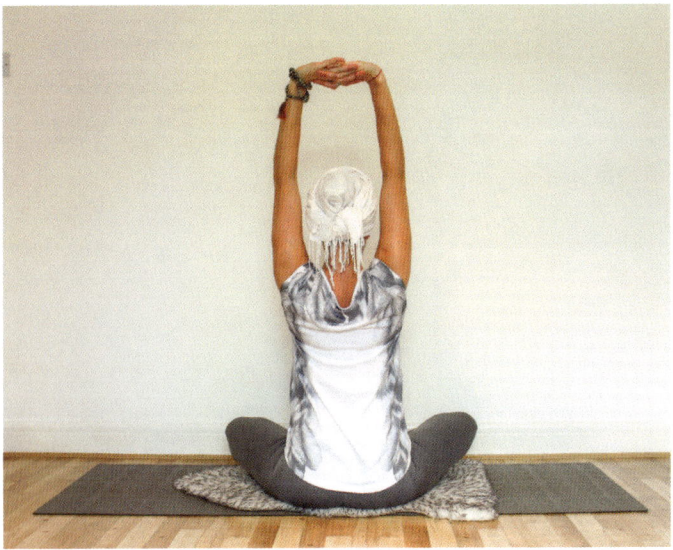

5. Arm Pumps Up 2-3 Minutes

Instructions: Still sitting, interlace your fingers behind the head, palms up. From there, inhale as you stretch the arms up and exhale back to the original position. Continue rapidly, inhaling up, exhaling down.

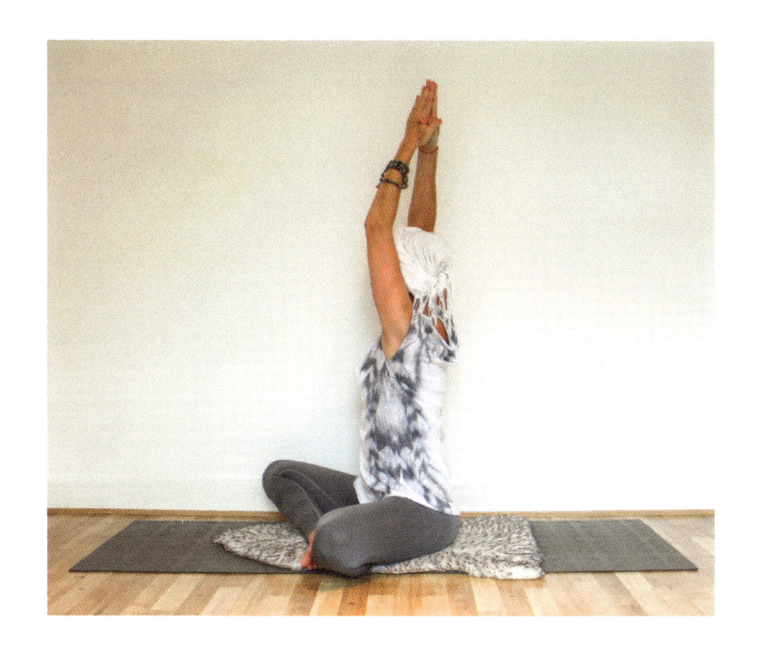

6. Torso Twists 2-3 Minutes

Instructions: Immediately stretch the arms up in prayer above the head. Cross your thumbs to help hold the position. Then inhale as you twist the torso to the left, exhale as you twist right.

To End: Inhale in the centre, hold and apply Mula Bandha.

Benefits: This is a detoxifying and strengthening exercise for the lungs.

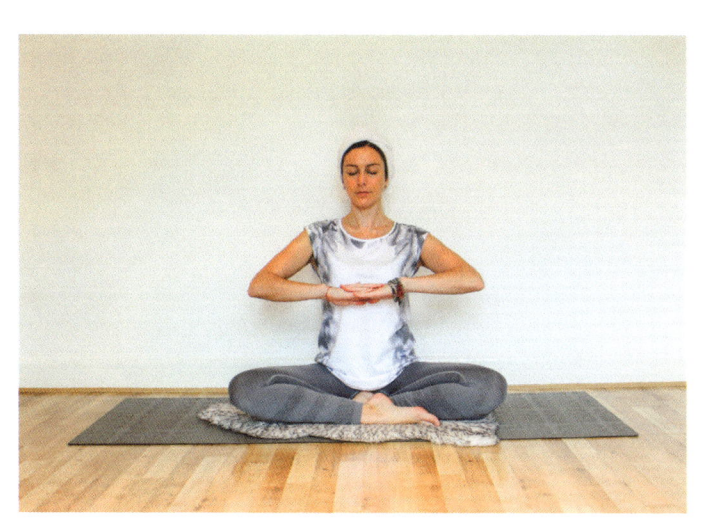

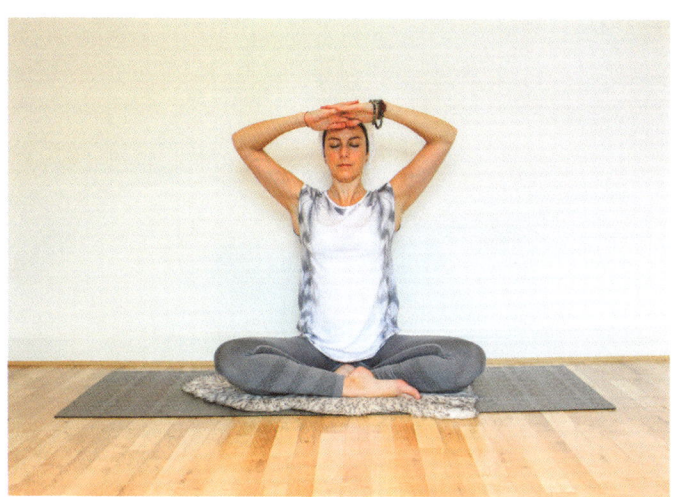

7. Heart Pumps 2-3 Minutes

Instructions: Sitting, interlace the fingers, thumbs touching, palms down in front of the heart. As you inhale, draw the hands up to the Third Eye at the forehead, then exhale back down to the heart. Continue rapidly with a strong breath.

To End: Inhale and hold for 10-15 seconds.

Benefits: I like to think of this exercise as drawing all those unnecessary thoughts from the head down into the heart, working to create compassion and ease.

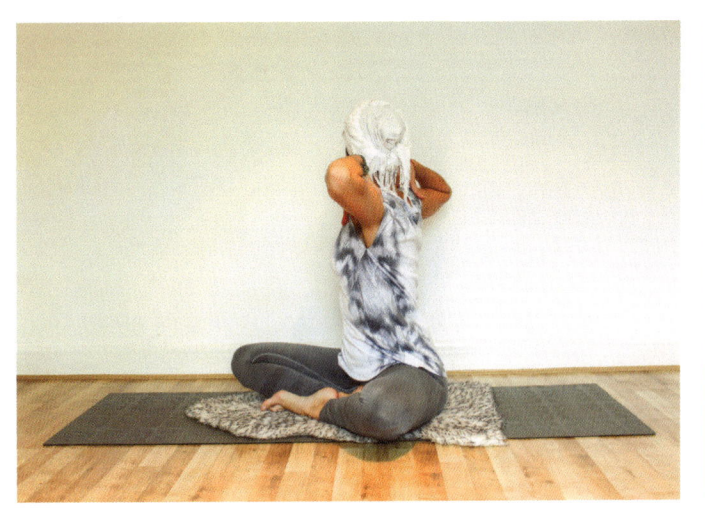

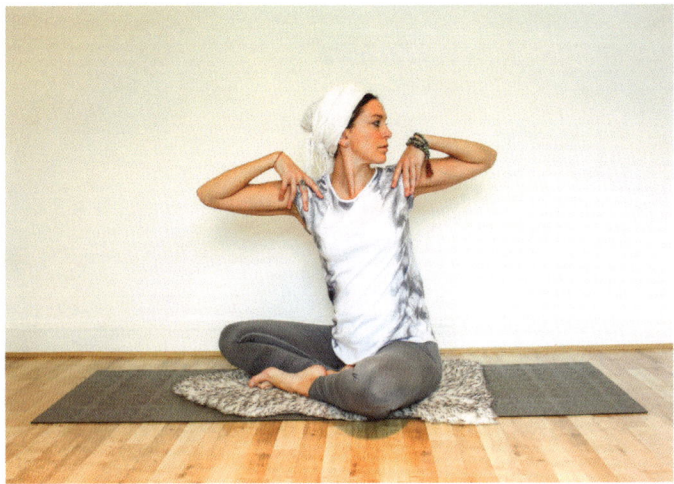

8. Spinal Twists 2-3 Minutes

Instructions: Take hold of your shoulders, fingers in front, thumbs behind, elbows up in line with the shoulders. Then inhale and twist to the left, exhale and twist right. Let the head follow the heart – don't hold your neck rigid.

To End: Inhale in the centre, hold and apply Mula Bandha for 10-15 seconds.

Benefits: This opens the lungs, brings flexibility to the spine and is detoxifying.

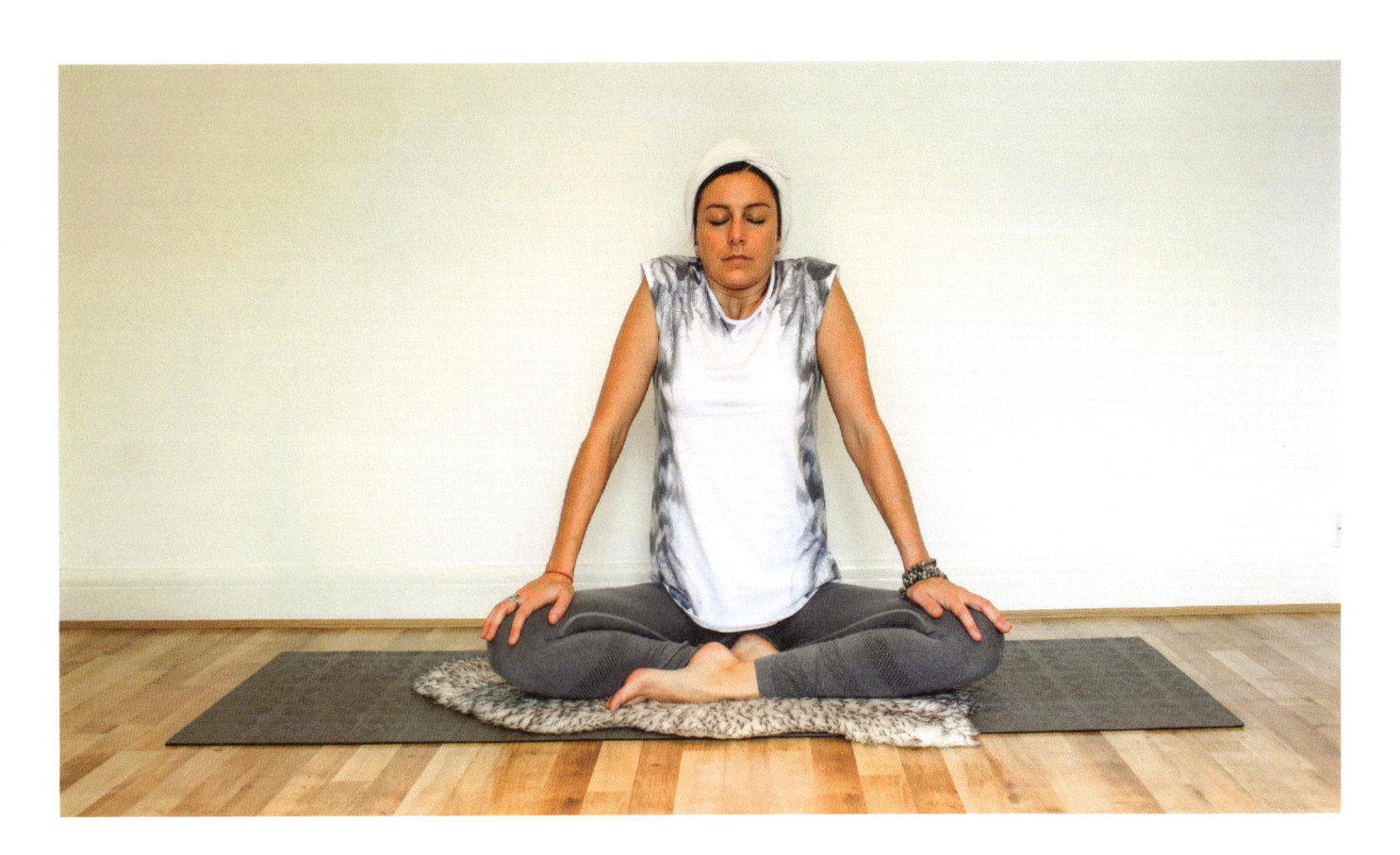

9. Shoulder Shrugs 2-3 Minutes

Instructions: Sitting tall, inhale as you raise both shoulders then exhale and drop them down and continue at a quick, steady pace.

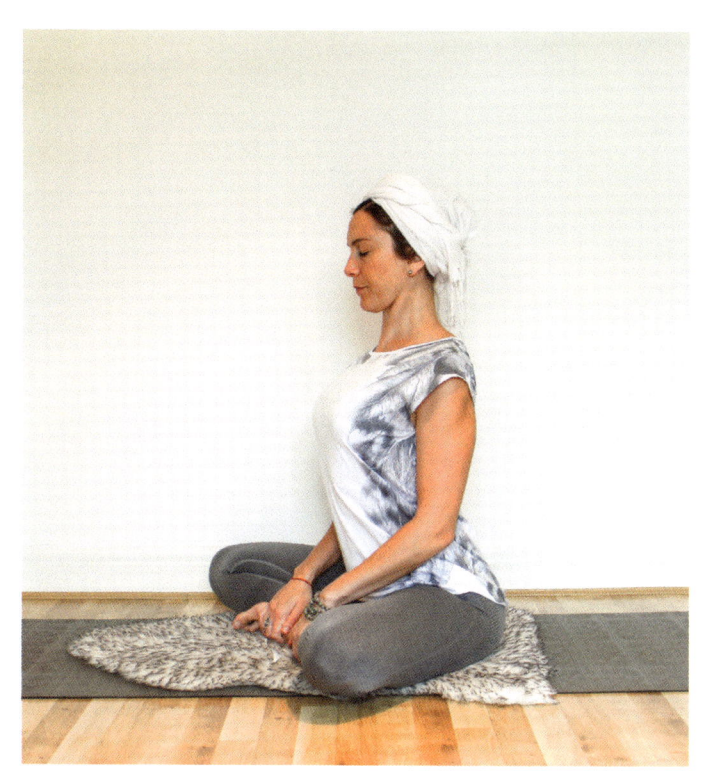

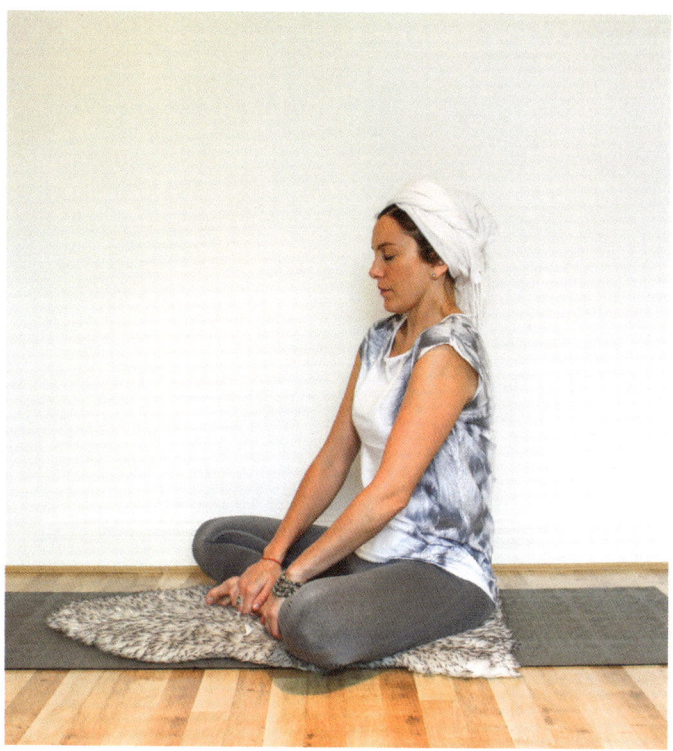

10. Spinal Flex 2-3 Minutes

Instructions: Sitting tall, keeping your head in line with the base of the spine, inhale as you draw the torso forward (opening the chest and pulling the shoulders back), then exhale and round the spine.

11. Meditation Next Page

The meditation, listed next, is the final part of this Kriya. Go straight into it.

DEEP MEDITATION

POSITION

Sitting tall with closed eyes, roll your vision up as if you're looking out of the top of your head.

Simply breathe long and deep in this position.

The key is to keep your eyes rolled up.

DURATION

15 Minutes

COMMENTS

This is a brilliant meditation for beginners when combined with the preceding kriya.

#embodyyoursoulpurpose

@roisinallanakiernan

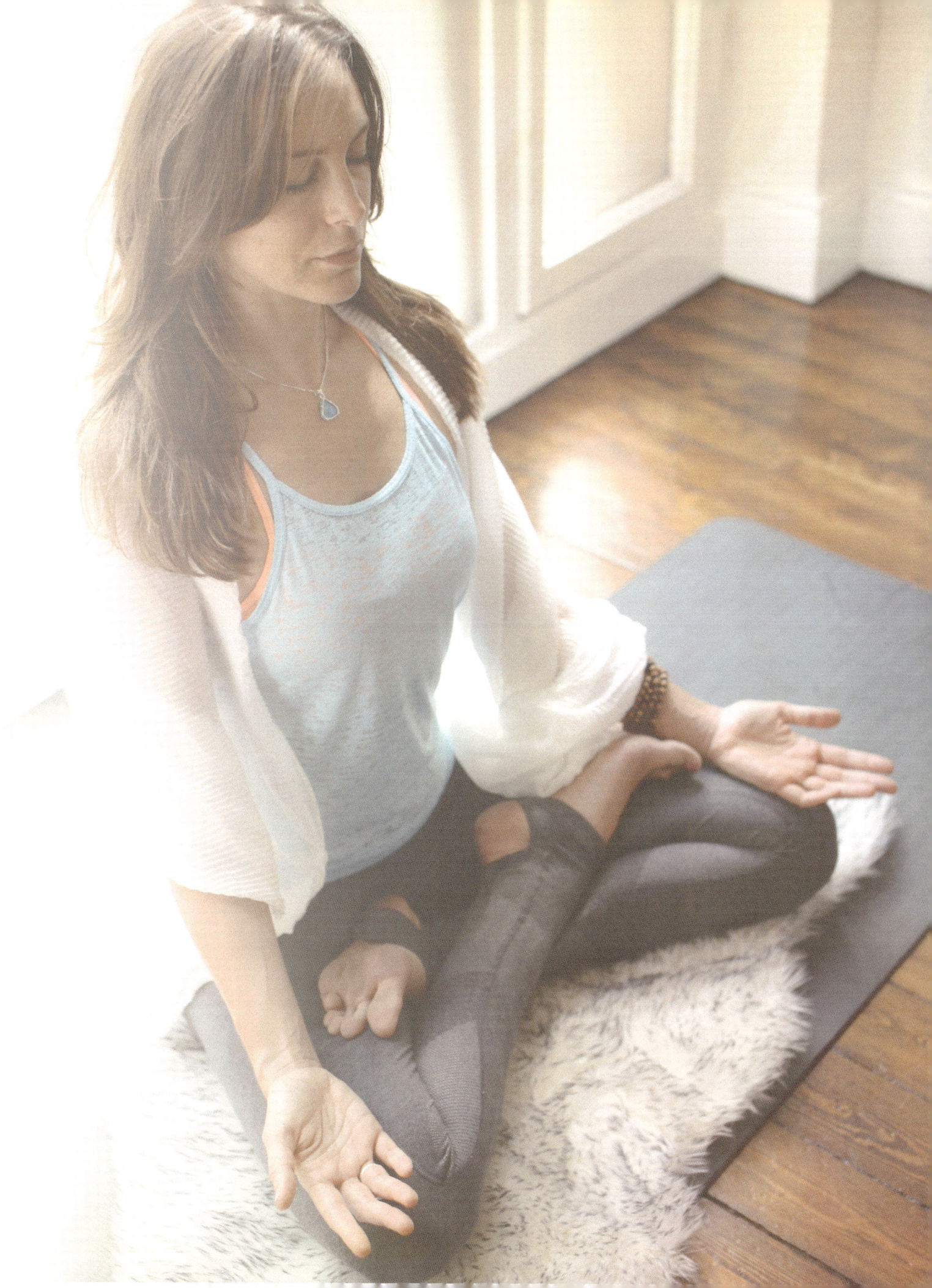

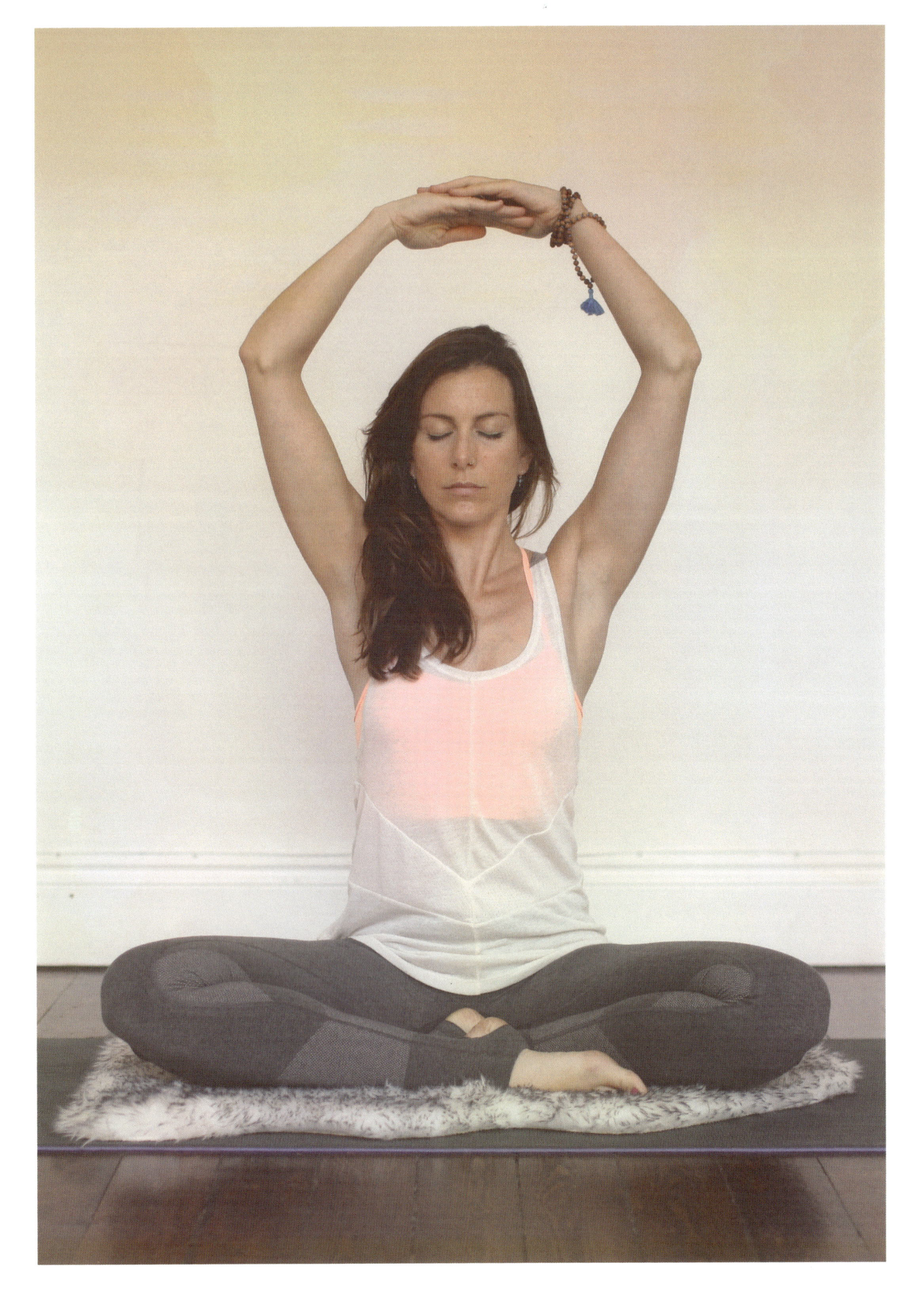

9

THE SUBTLE BODY

MYSTERY OR MASTERY

Go deep into the core of you by staying put and focussing with discernment, discipline and patience. In this way you can choose mastery over your life, rather than circling the mystery.

#embodyyoursoulpurpose
@roisinallanakiernan

THE SUBTLE BODY
MYSTERY OR MASTERY

It is through the ninth, Subtle Body that you're given an opportunity to master your essence, your true self.

The Subtle Body is your Soul's carriage (it holds the Akashic Records, the wisdom of your previous lifetimes) taking your essence through the cycles of life - between death and rebirth. That said, the Subtle Body in this lifetime requires that you stay put. Constantly moving or changing focus will make your energy scattered and exacerbate the mystery of life. To stay put requires discipline and patience and offers an opportunity to go deep into your core – an opportunity to master you.

In this Subtle Body, we can either circle the mystery of life, or choose mastery.

Being so close to 10 – to the completion of the soul's journey - can bring about a desire for perfection, which, on the one hand, provides a sense of direction but can also create frustration. In turn, this frustration can make you clutch at threads, scattered in energy, aggressive, insecure and overfocussed on the end goal. A lack of focus can also create a desire for stimulants.

Having got this far you could become obsessed with the end goal and forget the journey you've had and are still having. You could forget that others are on their own personal journey too and get frustrated with them. You could become demanding of others, wanting to manage them in order to gain focus in yourself.

Alternatively, you could stay put, truly focus on yourself, your home and craft, and refine yourself. This is where the real joy of the Subtle Body comes into action - by letting go of the end goal and simply enjoying the journey with focussed direction. In this way you can find peace in the present moment. You can also learn to trust in the process of the journey, let go of scattered thoughts about what you feel you should be doing and simply concentrate on the task at hand in each moment. This is exemplary of the state of peaceful contentment that can be found in mastering the Subtle Body.

It is in staying put that you realise the law of cause and effect, because all will come to you – you have only to focus and let go and all you need for your journey will come. Again, this shows the difference between clutching at scattered threads and holding a clear focus.

In being subtle, you'll become aware of all the elements of life; all the bodies and their differing energies. This will also help with refining your goals. In harnessing the discernment, care and awareness of the Subtle Body, you can create an integral sense of self –one that surrenders to the collective consciousness whilst maintaining integrity in its own goals and sense of self.

By trusting in the process or journey and recognising the bigger picture that's at play you can find peace, relinquishing your individual need for control and surrendering into the collective consciousness, thereby accelerating the completion of your Soul's (1) individual journey in the Radiant Body's (10) wholeness.

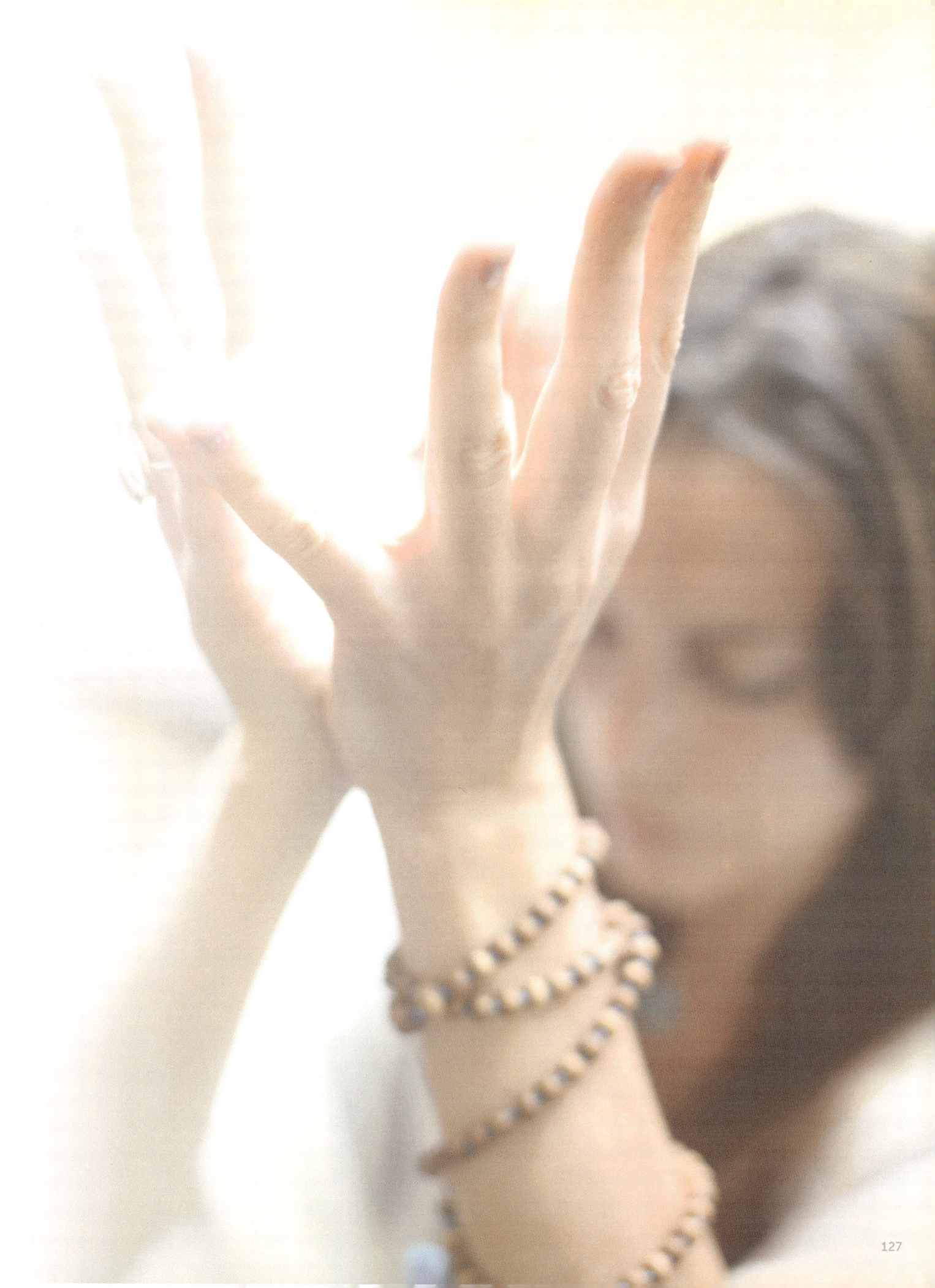

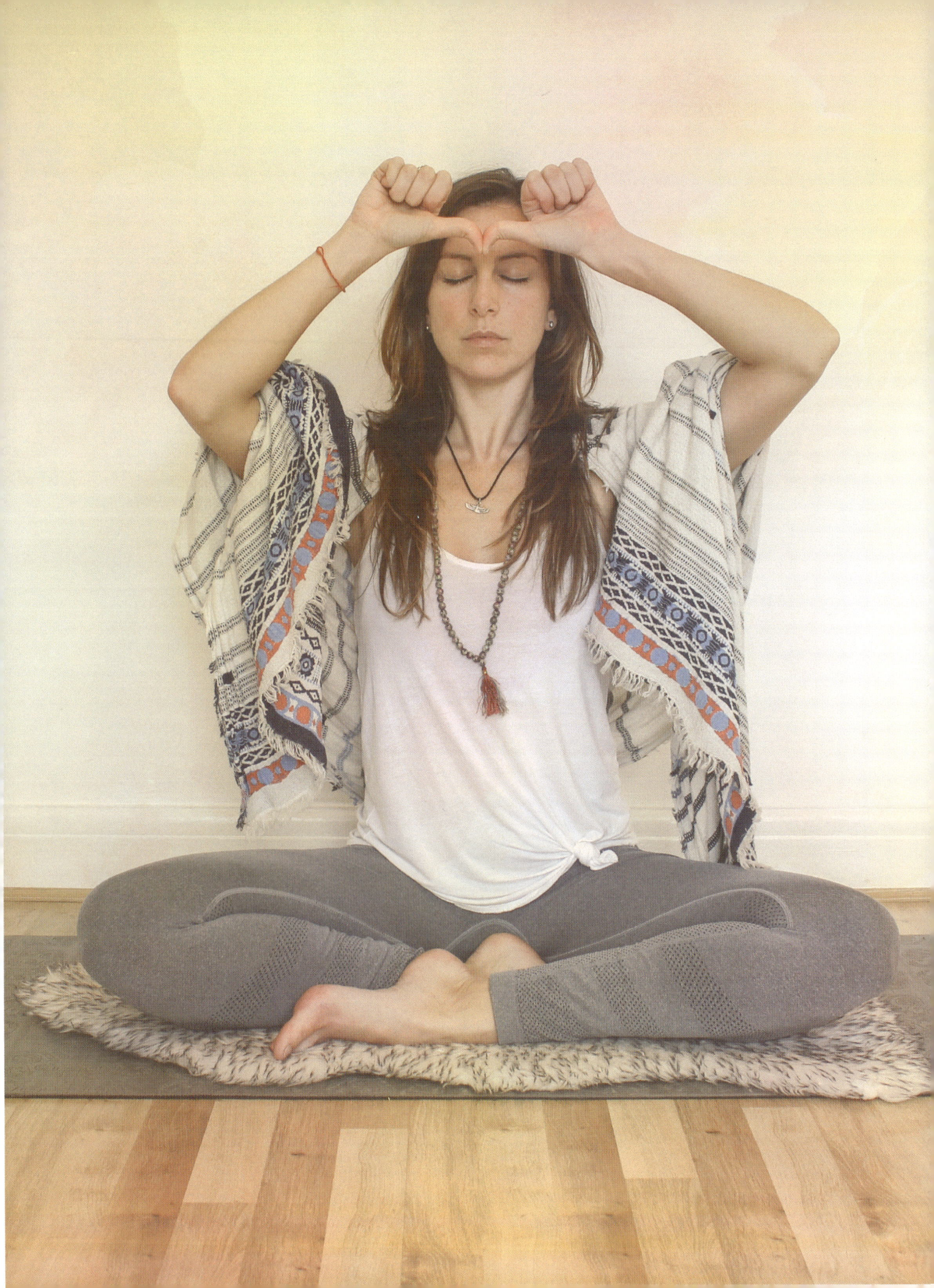

PRANAYAMA

MEDITATION ON THE WHITE SWAN

POSITION

Sit with a tall spine and bring your hands into fists. The thumbs extend out with the tips touching - press firmly so the thumb tips go white.

Don't push too hard on the thumb tips – just enough. It's important to relax your thumb joints – let them bend but don't force.

With the hands in this way, bring your thumb tips up in line with your eyes. Get a clear mental image of that part of your hands then close the eyes and 'look', mentally, at the thumb tips through closed eyes.

Breathe long and deep, mentally chanting 'Sat' on the inhale and 'Nam' on the exhale.

MANTRA

Sat Nam
(Truth is my identity)

DURATION

5 - 11 Minutes

COMMENTS

This meditation brings the experience and potential of many lives. It's one of the most sacred and secret meditations practised by the early Christians.

The thumb tips connect to the lung meridian and grief that may be held in the heart. In this respect, the meditation is especially good for childhood grief - in releasing pent up pain and helping you to 'stay put', feel more and move through it.

After 3 – 5 minutes you should feel locked into the position – you'll totally relax into it, with the arms supporting themselves. A feeling of ease will descend throughout your whole body, whilst the position will work to continuously stimulate the life nerves. Soon after your brain will relax and you'll start to 'float' in the mental realm.

The arch of the thumbs look like a swan's neck and represent your inner grace, bringing through the neutral mind; the Sattva Guru (purity) within.

Start slowly with it – about 5 minutes at a time – and gradually increase. This is a good meditation to practise before bed - 11 minutes is best at this time.

#embodyyoursoulpurpose
@roisinallanakiernan

KRIYA 1

TO CLARIFY THE SUBTLE BODY

This meditation works to clarify The Subtle Body's ability to attract opportunities. It also strengthens the Arcline.

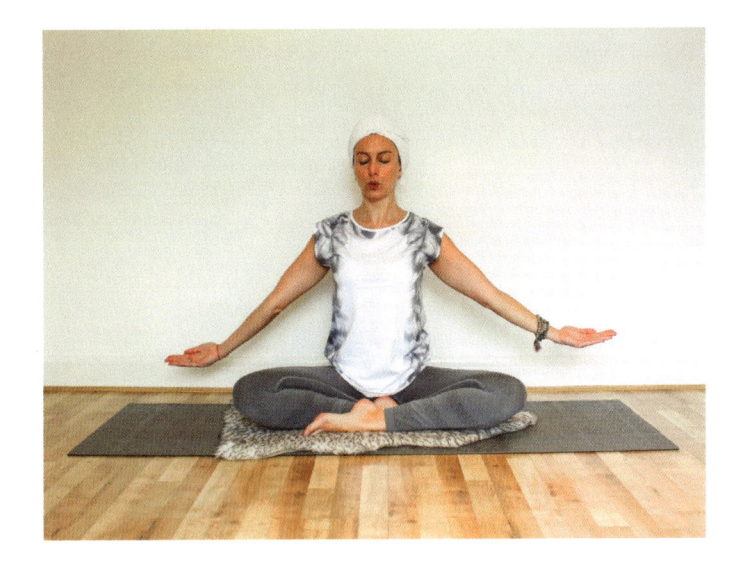

1. Clarify The Subtle Body
Begin With 11 Minutes

Instructions: Sit with a tall spine, chin in and chest out. Then place your arms by your sides but not touching the floor – your palms face upwards. Keeping your hands in this way, move your arms up so that the left palm overlaps the right a few inches above the head. The thumbs do not touch.

Mantra: Use the 'Tantric Har' recording to move with; a rhythm of about one second per 'Har'.

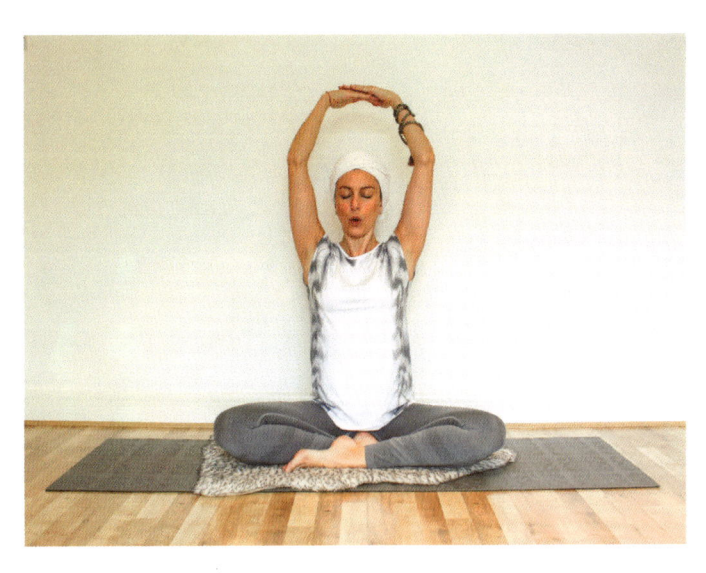

Har

On one 'Har', as you inhale through your mouth, raise your hands to the overhead position. Then, on the next 'Har', as you exhale though the mouth, release your hands to the start position. And continue in this way. Use the navel to bring some power to your breathing..

To end, interlace your fingers above your head with straight arms. Inhale and hold as you stretch through the whole body for 10-15 seconds then exhale. Repeat two more times.

"Do it just eleven minutes, you will start spacing out, so don't do more than eleven minutes when you get perfectly done and then you do it for twenty minutes, twenty two minutes and maximum you can do thirty three minutes in your lifetime. That's the max in it. And you cannot believe where you will stand, you will be so bright and shiny, people will not be in a position to look at your face. Aha, I am not kidding. It's very, very simple."

Yogi Bhajan – October 11, 1996

KRIYA 2

LAYA YOGA - FOR INTUITION AND THE POWER TO HEAL

This Kriya is key to opening the subtle realms of creative sound or Naad – the magic of mantra. By dropping into the sounds of this mantra, following it as it weaves through your body, you'll find yourself merging with the vastness of your Higher Self – strengthening your intuition and giving you the power to heal.

The mantra works with three and a half cycles - the pulse rhythm of the Kundalini energy, which is often represented as being coiled three and a half times. In this way, it works to directly awaken the Kundalini force, connecting you with all of creation and empowering you to sense your more subtle bodies.

'Laya' means to suspend from the ordinary world. This kriya, therefore, helps you to step beyond the base nature of existence and fixes your attention on a higher state of consciousness. It lets you absorb the bliss of infinite vastness, awakening you to a different state of being – one without distractions and attachments and reactions from such.

Practising this for 40-120 days will etch your connection to the Infinite into your subconscious, offering liberation into your true identity.

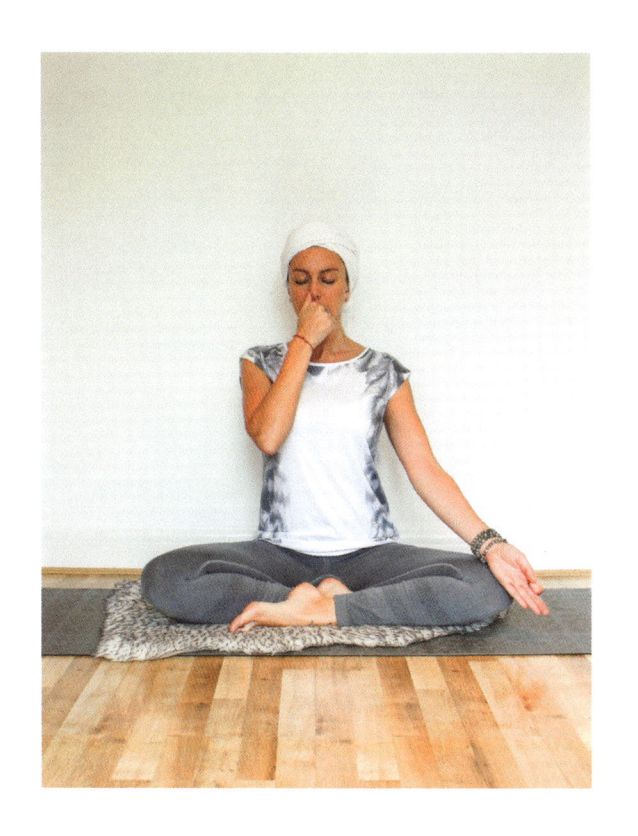

1. Nostril Breathing (Both Sides)

2-3 Minutes

Instructions: Sit with a tall spine and gently pull Mula Bandha (Root Lock) and Jalandhar Bandha (Neck Lock). Rest your left hand in Gyan Mudra (index finger touching thumb) in your lap and use your right hand to block the right nostril. Close the eyes and focus at the Third Eye (in and up between the brows). Then breathe long and deep through the left nostril.

As you breathe, visualise each area of the body – from the top of the head to the tips of the toes – and draw your breath to each and every part; allowing the prana (life force or breath) to circulate and revitalise each area.

To End: After completing each side, inhale deeply, hold briefly, then relax.

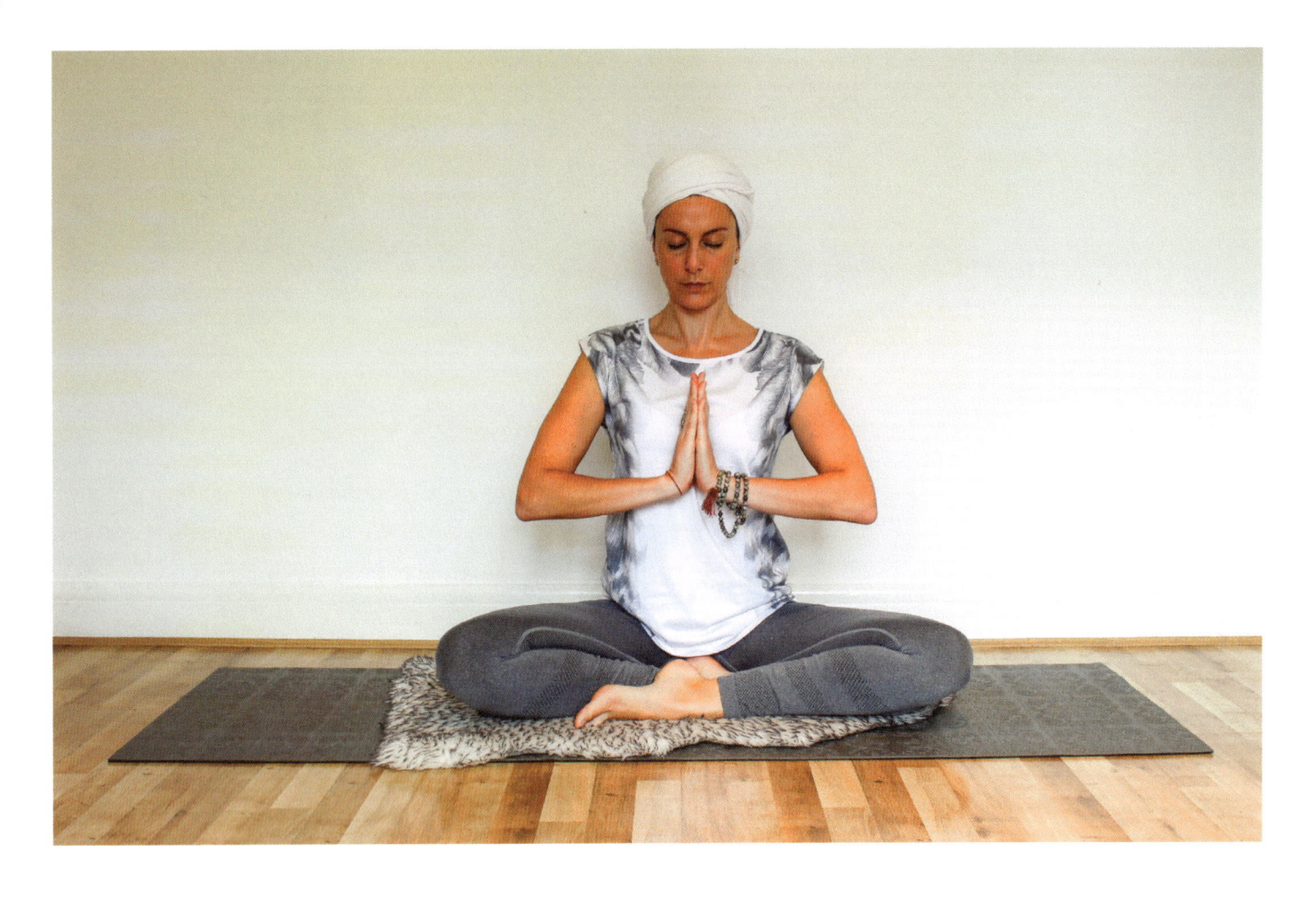

2. Prayer Mudra   LDB 2 Minutes / BOF 1 Minute

Instructions: Sitting with a straight spine, bring your hands together in prayer in the middle of the chest. Create a slight pressure between the hands and push the hands against the sternum, where the ribs meet at the base. Breathe long and deep (LDB) for 2 minutes.

Then begin (BOF) Breath of Fire (rapidly breathing in and out through the nostrils using the navel as a pump) for 1 minute.

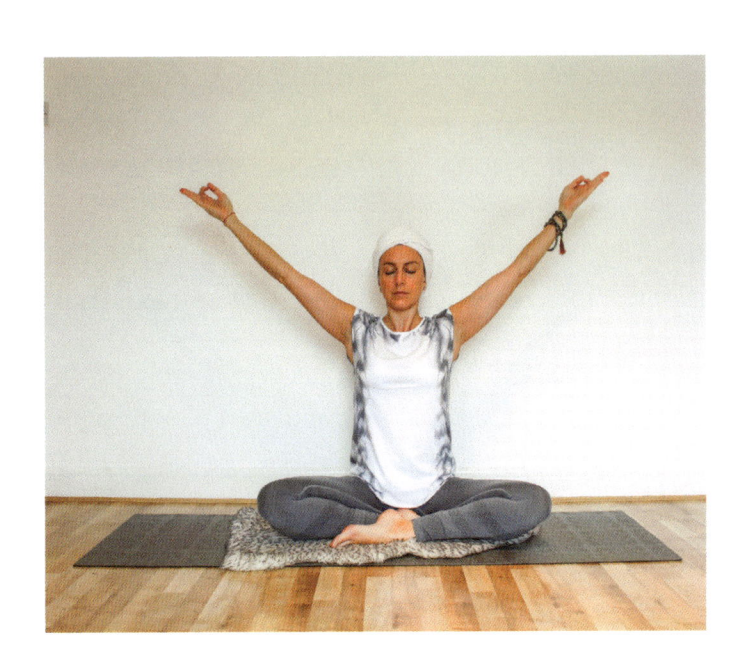

3. Arms Up in Gyan Mudra   3 Minutes

Instructions: Still sitting, bring your arms up at the sides, sixty degrees above your head. The palms face up towards the ceiling in Gyan Mudra (index fingers touching thumbs). Keep your arms straight, hold the position and breathe long and deep.

To End: Inhale and hold before relaxing.

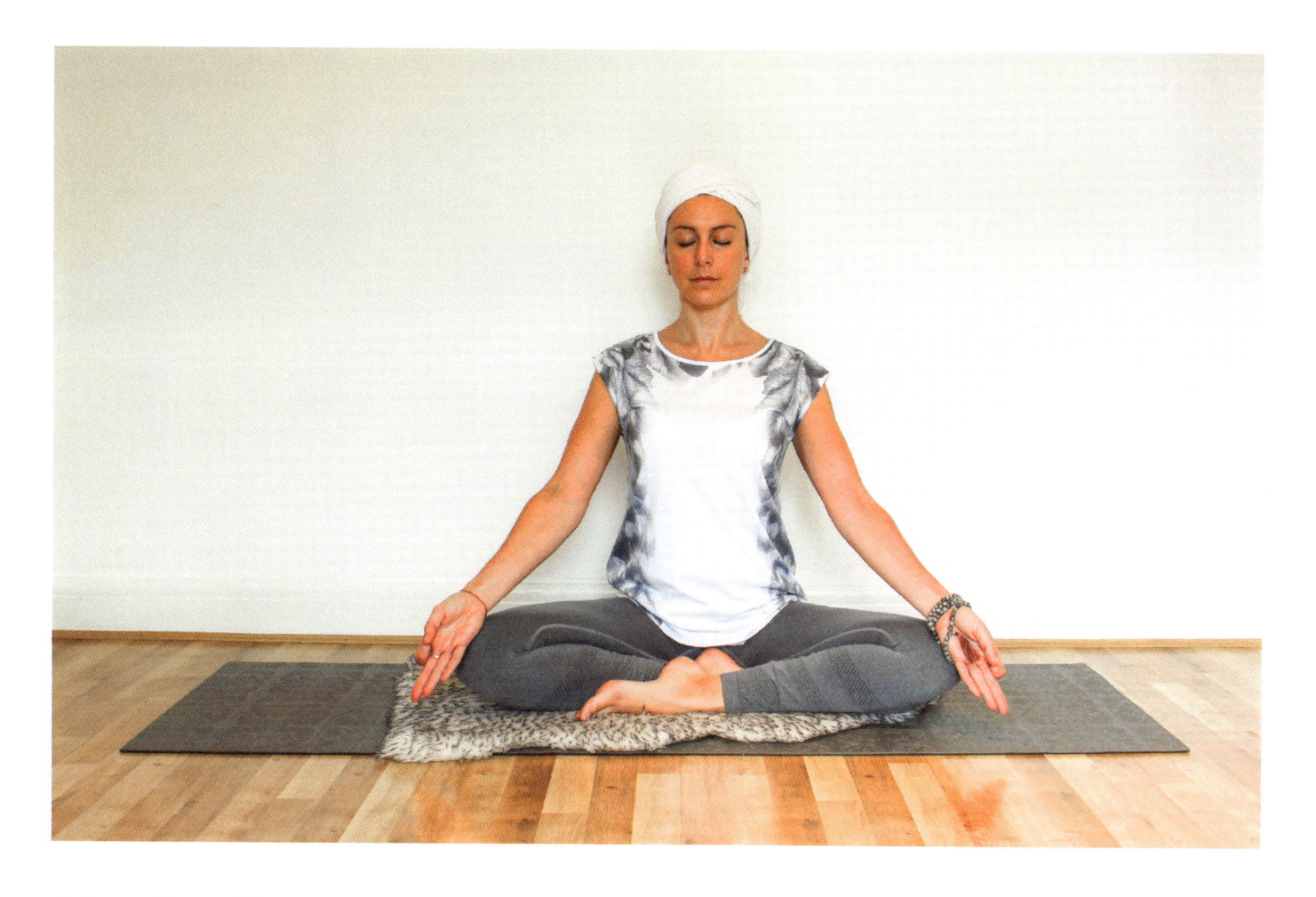

4. Laya Yoga Chant 11-31 Minutes

Instructions: Sit with a tall spine, arms straight and the hands on the knees in Gyan Mudra (index fingers touching thumbs).

We're going to chant a three and a half cycle mantra, which is the same rhythm as the flow of the Kundalini energy. So, as you chant, imagine it spiralling up from the base of your spine to the top of your head.

The Mantra:

Ek Ong Kar (uh)
Sa Ta Na Ma (uh)
Siree Wha (uh)
Hay Guru

Holding a light Mula Bandha (root lock) and Jalandhar Bandha (neck lock) you're going to chant in the following manner. On 'Ek' pull the navel in and on each 'uh' lift the diaphragm up firmly. The 'uh' is more of a powerful movement than a sound. When it comes to 'Hay Guru' relax the navel and abdomen.

The eyes are nine tenths closed and your attention is at the Third Eye.

To End: Inhale deeply and hold the breath as long as you can before exhaling and relaxing.

MEDITATION

ANTAR NAAD MUDRA

POSITION

Sitting with a straight spine, bring the hands in prayer at the navel. You're going to raise your hands up from prayer at the navel and start opening them at the Heart Centre as you work your way to a full Lotus Mudra at the Third Eye, before turning the tops of the hands in on each other and drawing them back down through the middle to the start position.

DURATION

11 - 31 Minutes

MOVE WITH THE MANTRA

The first verse takes you to a Lotus Mudra at the Third Eye.

Sa Re Sa Sa,
Sa Re Sa Sa,
Sa Re Sa Sa,
Sa Rung

The second verse brings you back down through the middle to the starting position.

Har Re Har Har,
Har Re Har Har,
Har Re Har Har,
Ha Rung

#embodyyoursoulpurpose
@roisinallanakiernan

In full Lotus Mudra your palms are facing each other with the base of the hands, thumbs and baby fingers touching with the rest of the fingers spread open like a lotus flower.

The breath will find its own flow.

COMMENTS

This mantra connects to the etheric realm and helps to strengthen it within you, thereby strengthening your Subtle Body.

'Sa' is the Infinite totality, God/Ether (contains all).

'Har' is the creativity of the Earth; the finite manifestation of the divine in the personal.

'Ung' is the complete totality of infinite and finite.

It brings peace and prosperity, helping you conquer the wisdom of past, present, and future.

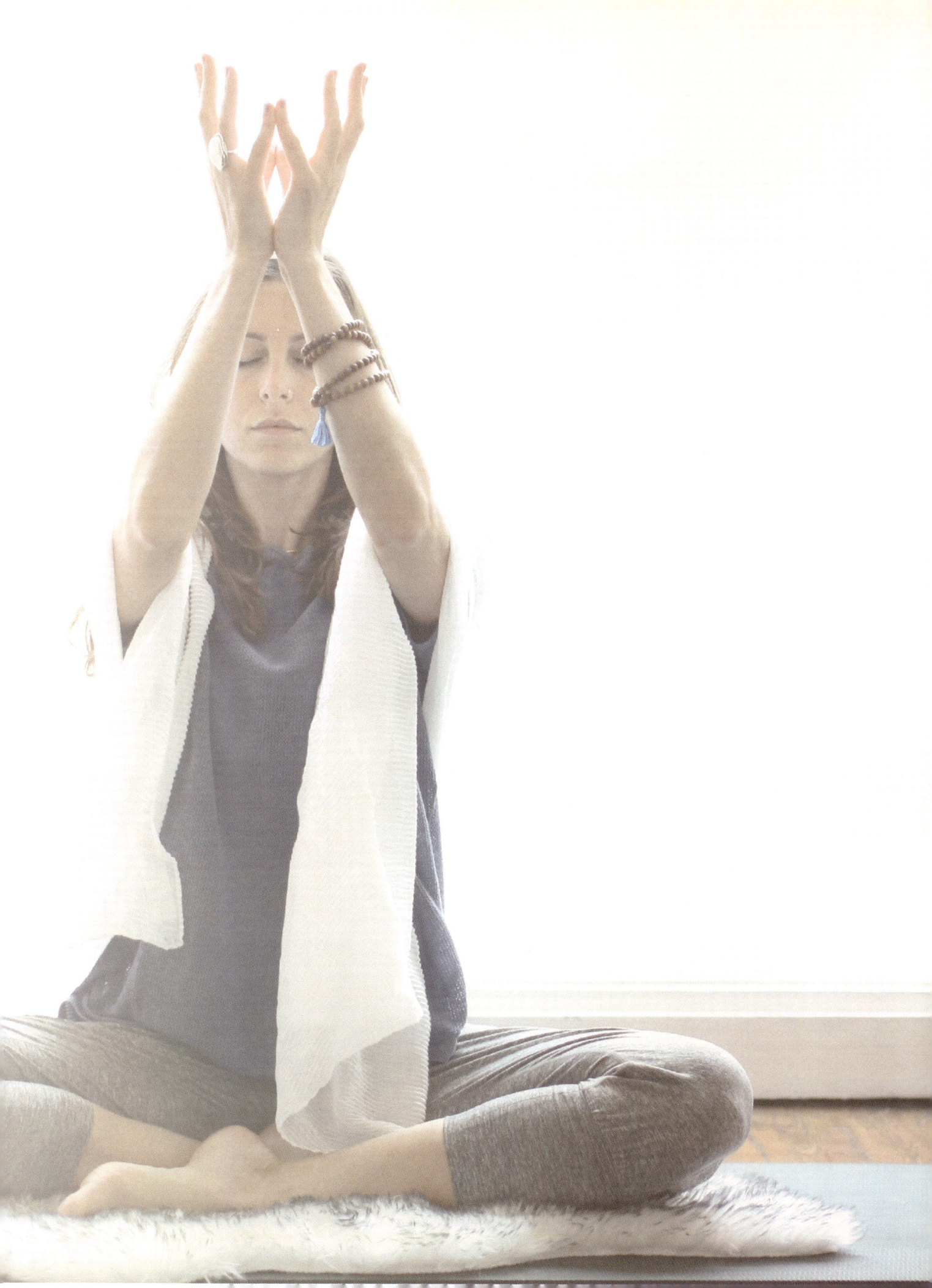

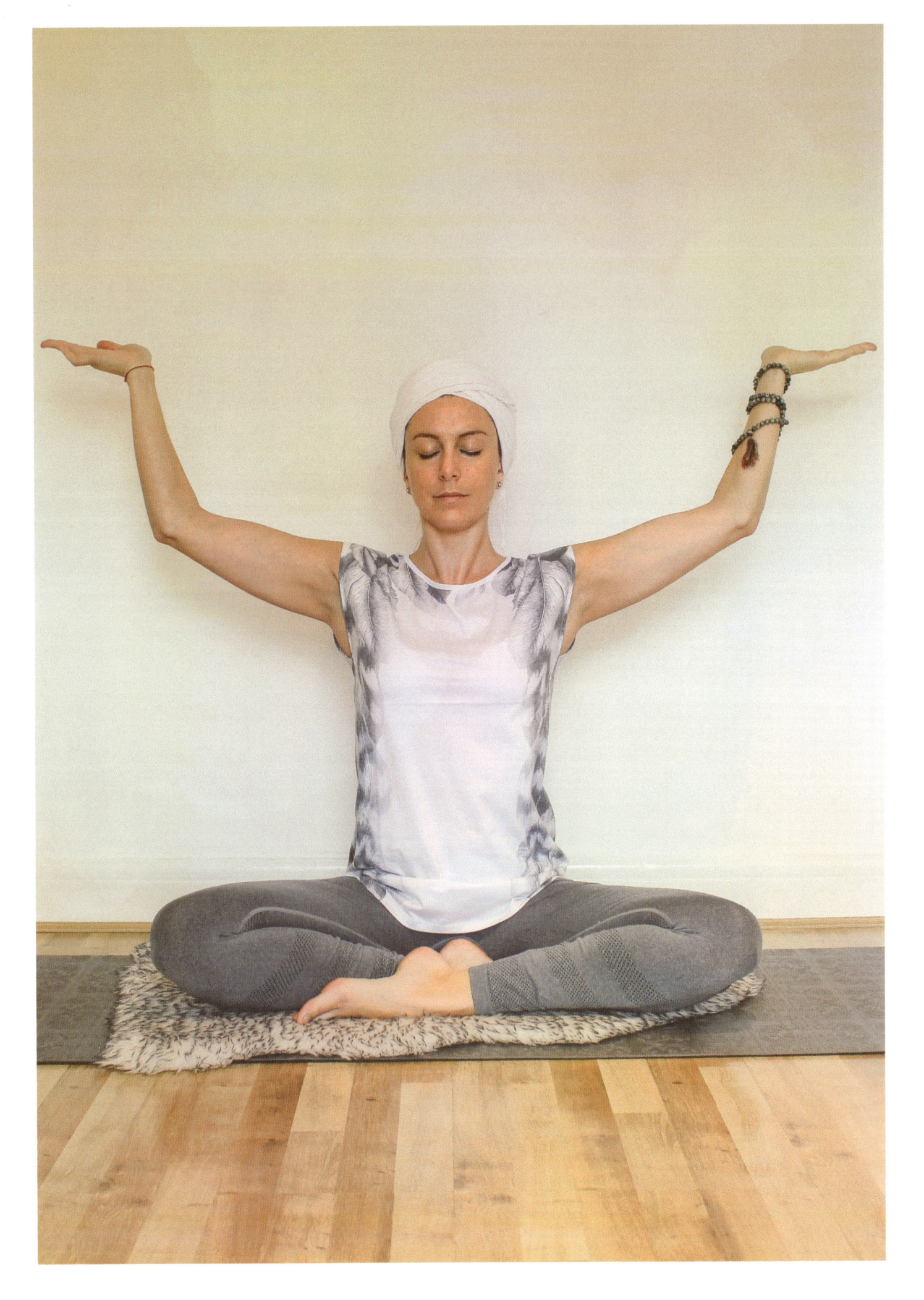

10

THE RADIANT BODY

ALL OR NOTHING

The combination of this 1 (Soul Body) with 0 can either offer infinite completion for the soul's journey or a removal of connection. You can either feel courageous or fearful; aspirational or unmotivated; confident or lacking self-esteem.

#embodyyoursoulpurpose
@roisinallanakiernan

THE RADIANT BODY
ALL OR NOTHING

The tenth, Radiant Body, being number 10, contains many of the qualities of the first, Soul Body (No.1), but the combination of this one with zero can either offer completion for the soul's journey or a removal of connection. The zero either enhances or nullifies the infinite connectedness of one - it's all or nothing.

In this position, your soul can either be realised or feel totally alone. You can either feel courageous or fearful; aspirational or unmotivated, confident or lacking self-esteem.

It is in these enemies of all or nothing that you'll feel the influence of five and ten – of the fifth and tenth bodies (the Physical and Radiant bodies). Through the fifth body you're shown the full soul story (your lessons needed for growth), whether you accept it or not. Then, through the tenth, you're given an opportunity to develop the courage to accept the implications raised in the fifth. It is through the fifth or the tenth that you can do or not, where you can take the lessons and act or not.

The tenth, Radiant Body, encompasses the 'royal self', not because of a realised individual self, but because of a surrender to the collective consciousness; because of the total abandonment of personal power. It is through this true, royal self, that you can activate dignity.

If 1, the soul, offers an opportunity for humility, then 10 provides the opportunity for total humility or, indeed, a total removal of any opposing feelings towards such.

The Tenth Gate, often thought of as the crown of the head, is the portal to The Divine. It is the same with the tenth, Radiant Body. By relinquishing any personal power, by uniting your individual will with the conscious collective, you can merge, in soul completion, with The Divine.

A strong Radiant Body will attract all you need and give you the courage to utilise it with dignity.

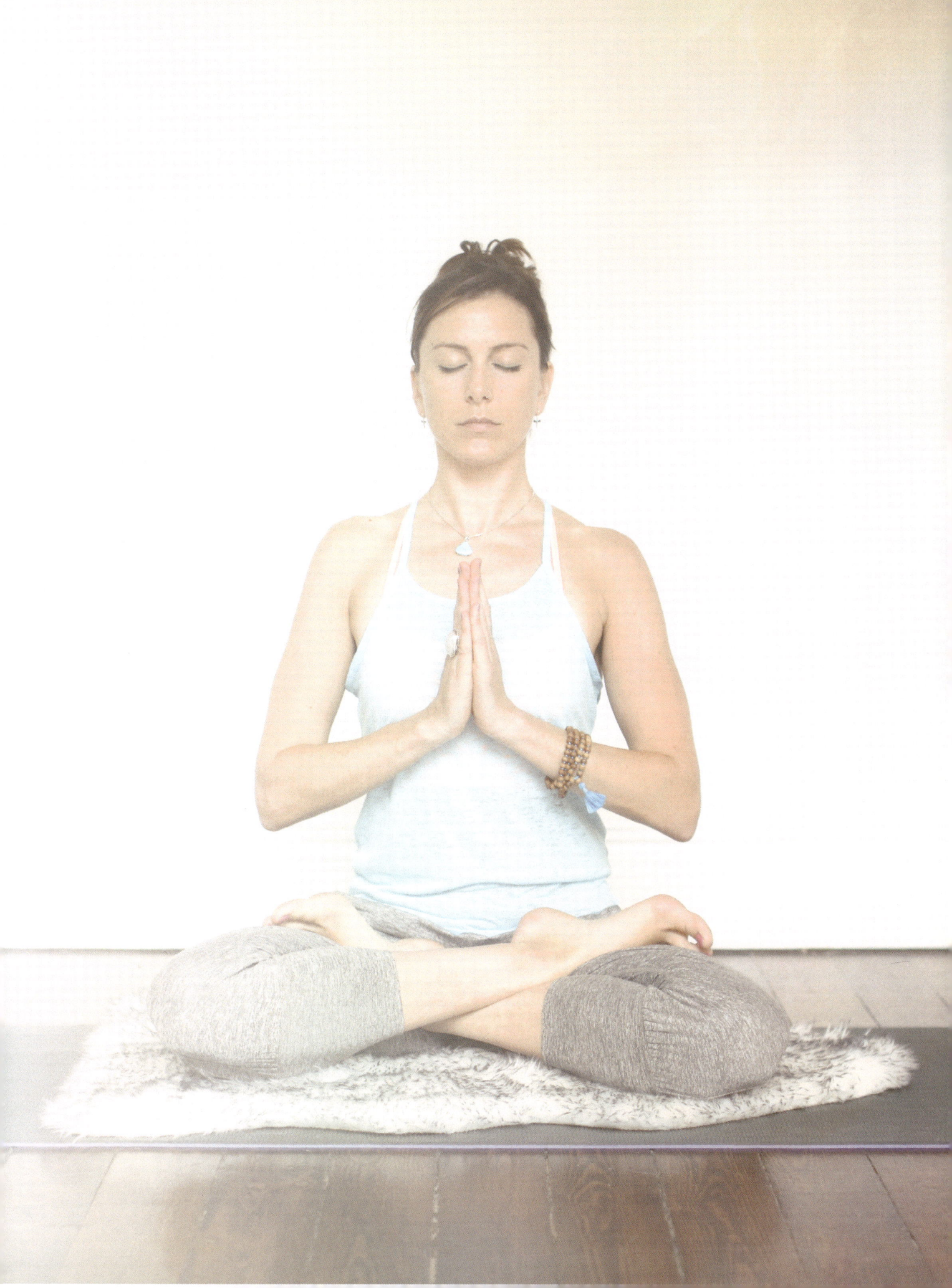

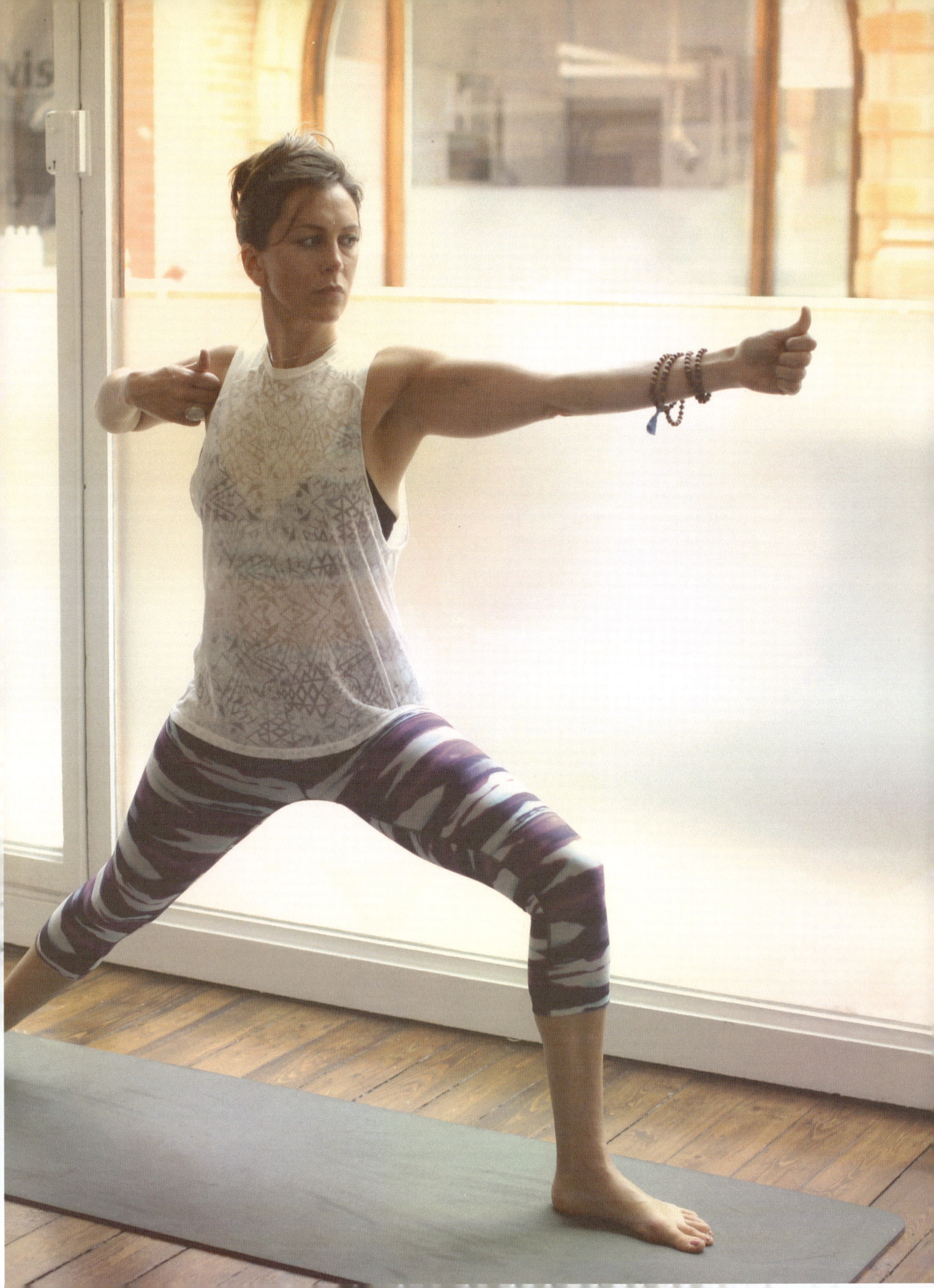

PRANAYAMA
ARCHER POSE (WARRIOR 2)

POSITION

Standing at the back of your mat, take a long step forward with your left leg. Turn the back, right foot out to support you and keep that leg straight. Then bend your left knee and bring it directly above the ankle.

Holding this position with the legs, reach back and take an imaginary bow and arrow from a bag at your back. Make fists with your hands but keep the thumbs up. Bring both hands in front of you, your left arm remains straight, holding the bow and your right hand pulls back to the shoulder with the arrow. Keep your right elbow bent up at the shoulder. Open your chest and look to your left thumb – to your focus.

Have the whole body engaged – this is a Warrior pose.

Hold and breathe long and deep.

Make sure you complete this on both sides.

DURATION

3 minutes minimum on each side.

Build it up, depending on level of fitness and the time you have to give it.

TO END

Inhale, pull the arrow back hard, re-focus your attention, hold the breath a moment and then shoot the arrow, stepping the feet together and resting a moment before completing the other side.

COMMENTS

This position develops confidence. It's a demanding position to hold, but with such a focus comes strength of spirit. When you break through your supposed limits in Kundalini, you break through so much more in life. In this way, you're able to hold yourself in any 'position' life throws at you, choosing to really feel each moment and act with courage and truth, without falling into habitual, reactionary patterns.

#embodyyoursoulpurpose
@roisinallanakiernan

KRIYA

FOR THE RADIANT BODY

This set develops the Spiritual Warrior within us - increasing the magnetism needed to draw in that which will support our growth, enabling us to see every situation as an opportunity, and giving us the courage to face life's seeming difficulties.

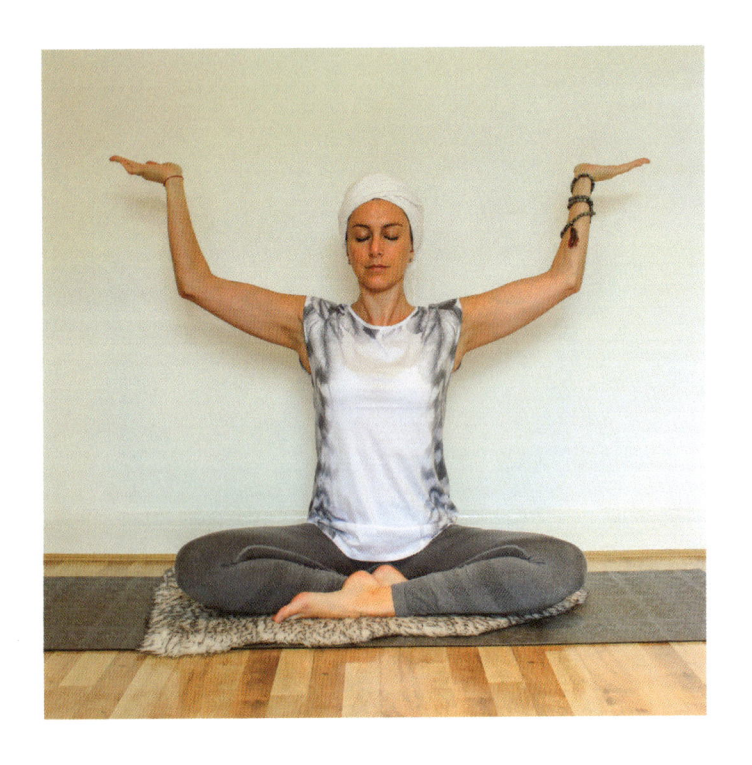

1. Arms Up And Open to Receive

1-3 Minutes

Instructions: Sitting tall, bring your arms out to the sides, bend the elbows and raise your forearms straight up, with the palms facing up. Hold this position, draw the navel in and breathe long and slow.

Benefits: This strengthens the arms and opens the chest.

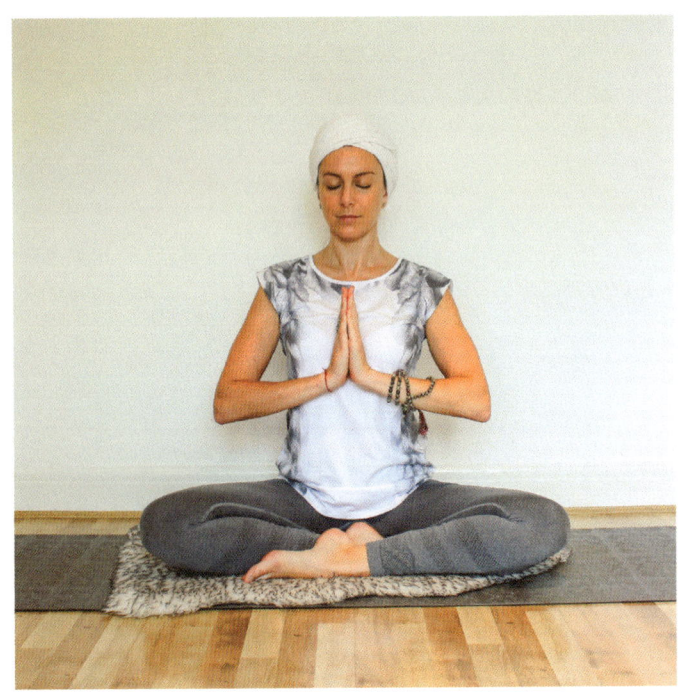

2. Sat Nam in Prayer Pose 1-3 Minutes

Instructions: Sitting tall, bring your hands into prayer in the middle of the chest. Holding this position, close the yes and chant Sat Nam (true name). Feel yourself becoming radiant – visualise light all around you.

Mantra:

Sat Nam

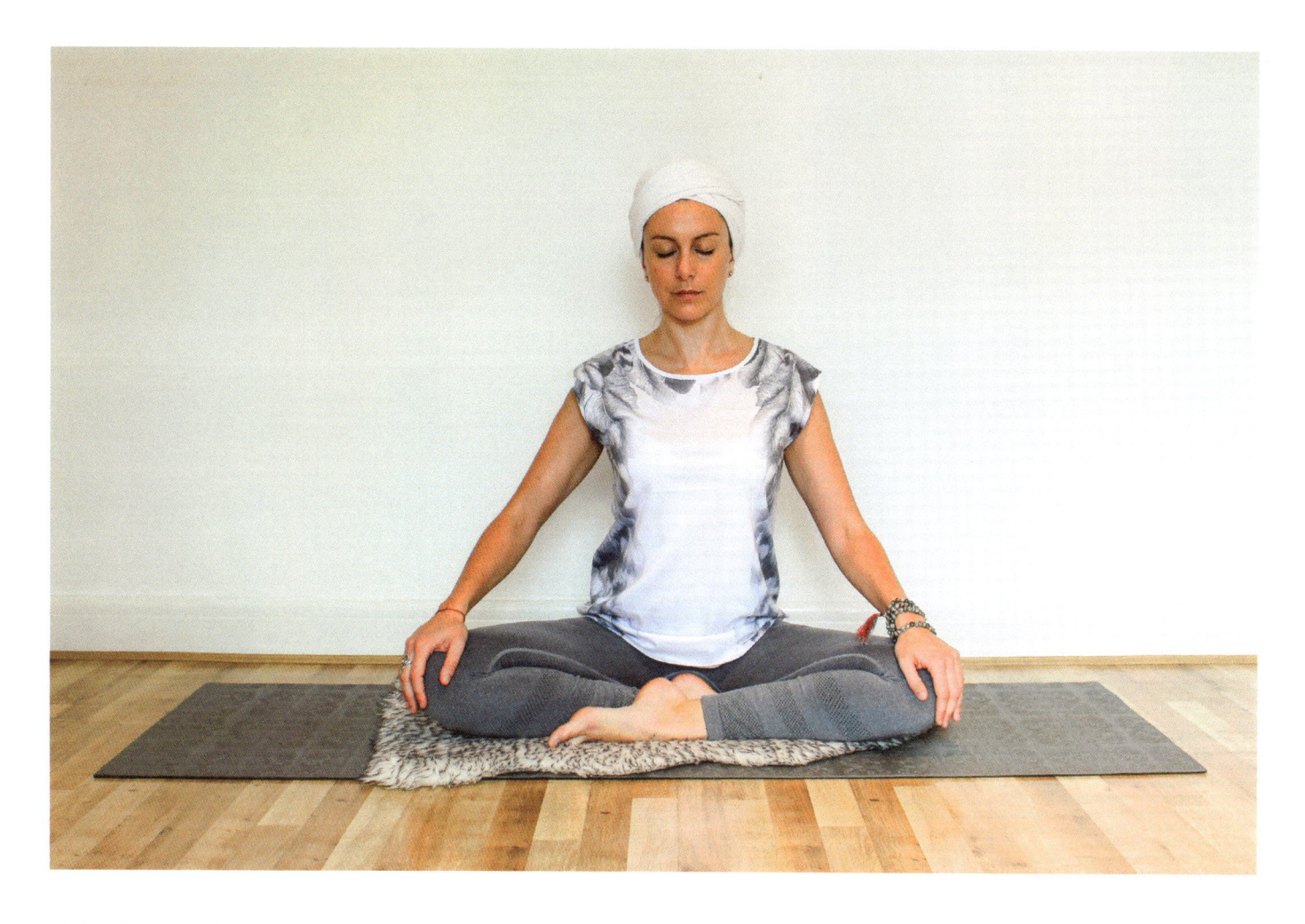

3. Sufi Grinds 1-3 Minutes In Both Directions

Instructions: Preferably sitting in Easy Pose (with crossed legs), take hold of your knees and inhale as you circle your upper body forward (opening the chest and shoulders as you go) and exhale (rounding the spine) as you circle back. Your shoulders stay in line with your hips; this is more of an internal movement. Do not move your head or neck. Feel yourself expanding from this heart centred position as you move.

Move in one direction and then switch to the other side – both for 1-3 minutes.

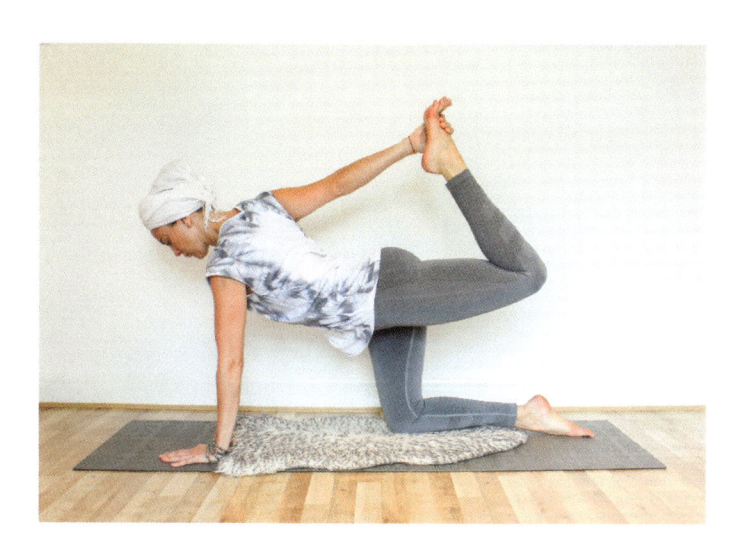

4. Bound Cow with Breath of Fire

1-3 Minutes On Both Sides

Instructions: Starting on your hands and knees, lift your left foot and take hold of it with your right hand. Stretch open as far as possible – use the leg to gently pull your shoulder open – then hold and use Breath of Fire (rapid inhale and exhale through the nose).

Benefits: Opens the shoulders, hips and abdominals, assisted also by the breath work.

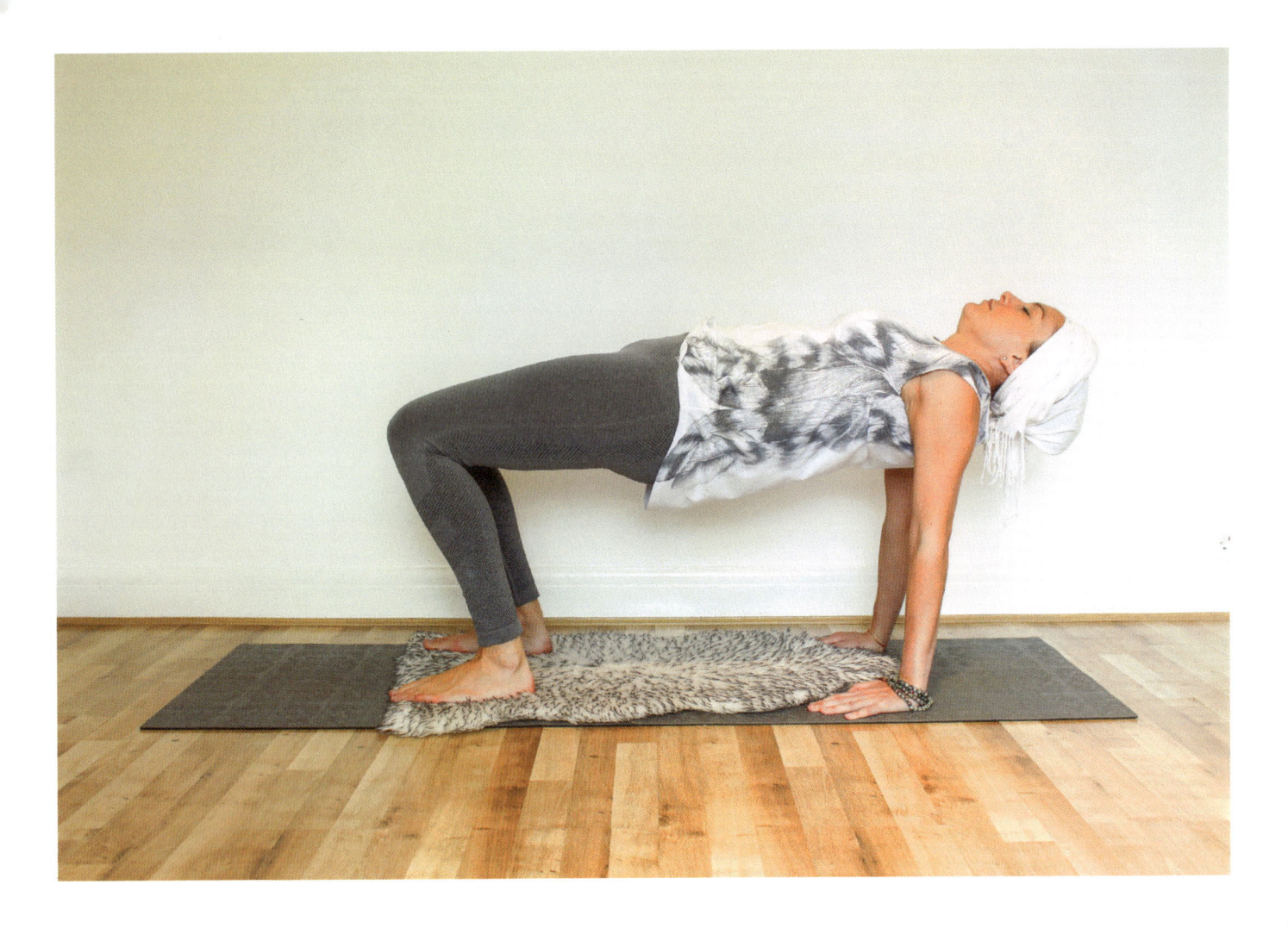

5. Bridge 1-3 Minutes

Instructions: Sitting tall with both legs extended and your hands flat on the floor beside you, bend the knees and bring your feet flat on the floor. Then, lift the hips as high as you can into Bridge Pose. Continue alternating between these positions – inhaling up and exhaling down.

Benefits: This pose rejuvenates body and mind through the circulatory increase along the spine and throughout the body.

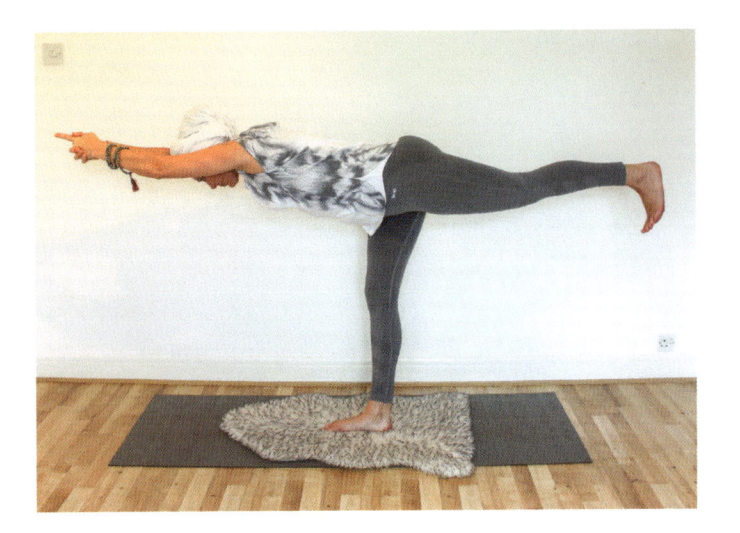

6. Warrior 3 1-3 Minutes

Instructions: Standing, interlace your fingers with the index fingers pointing up. Then, drawing your navel in and up to support the spine, push your right leg back, whilst hinging your upper body forward – so you create a 'T' shape with your body. Try to keep the hips square, use a flat foot to push back and reach forward with the fingers. Finding a point to focus on will help hold your balance. Breathing long will help steady you. Do not go over to the other side.

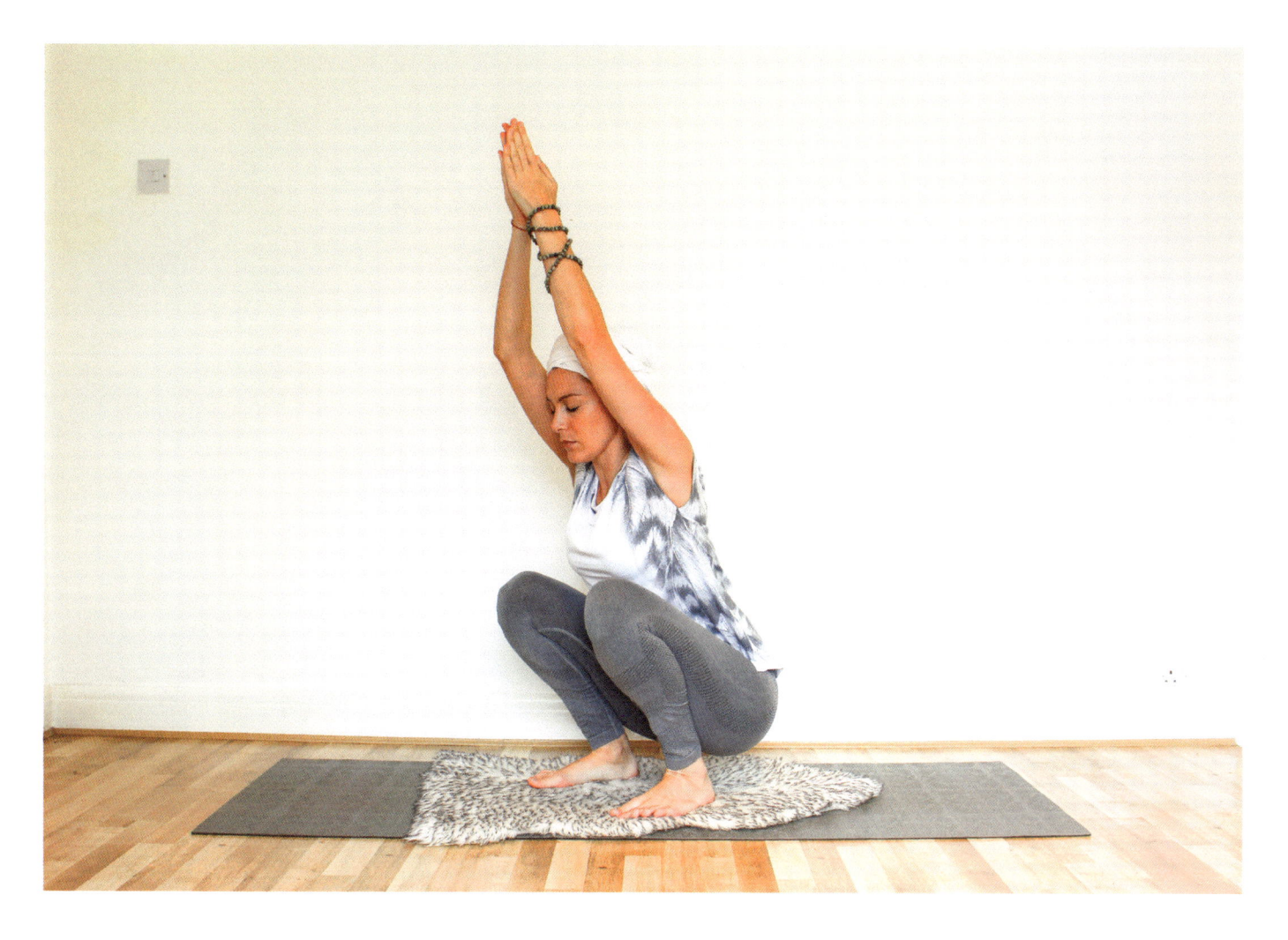

7. Crow Squats 1-3 Minutes

Instructions: Standing, feet hip distance apart and keeping your toes and knees facing forward, inhale as you sit down into a full deep squat bringing your arms up to prayer above then head. Then exhale back up, releasing your hands down by your sides. Continue alternating with these positions – inhaling down, arms up in prayer and exhaling up, arms down.

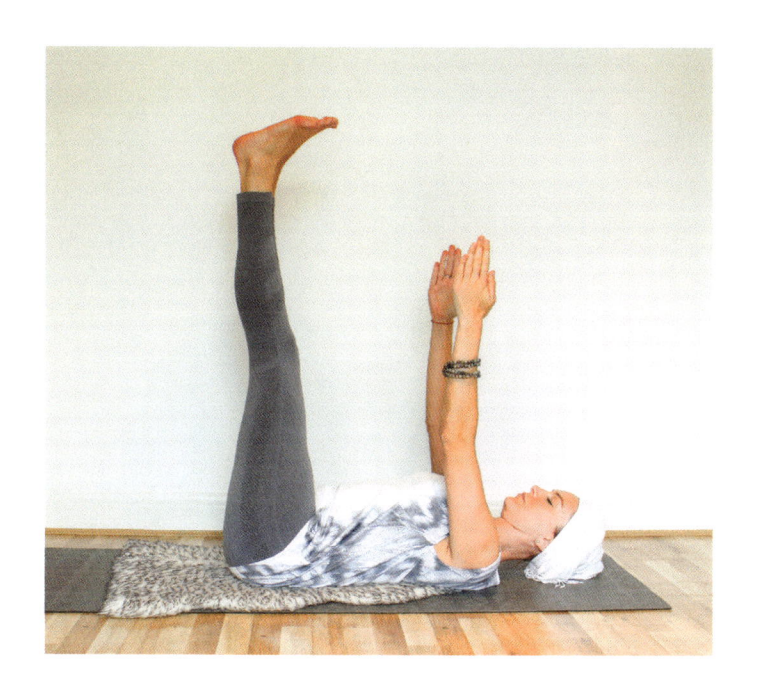

8. Legs Up 1-3 Minutes

Instructions: Lying on your back, bring your legs and arms up ninety degrees and hold. Feet are flat and hands are raised with the palms facing towards each other. Breathe long and deep.

Benefits: This is a strong but deeply relaxing exercise, stretching through the hamstrings and toning / engaging the abdominals whilst allowing the blood to be drawn back up to the heart.

MEDITATION
TO DEVELOP THE RADIANT BODY

POSITION

Sitting tall with a light Jalandhar Bandha (neck lock), arc your arms over the head, the fingers interlocked. Tuck your chin in and pull the arms back slightly.

Then, holding this position, with the eyes closed, chant the Ik Acharee Chand shabd - detailed below.

TO END

Keeping the position, inhale deeply, suspend the breath and stretch the arms up straight – the fingers remain interlaced. Exhale powerfully and repeat two more times. Then relax and shake out the arms.

MANTRA

COMMENTS

This is an extraordinary meditation, which should be practised with great precision. Make sure the hand mudra is held directly over the head. Also, as you chant, bring full awareness to every word – project and vibrate with them all as complete in themselves.

Teachers, this is an excellent meditation to assist you in holding the link and space for your students. Your communication will become impersonally personal; your hidden agendas will be put aside; and your presence will embody the teachings.

DURATION

11 - 22 minutes

Ajai Alai (Invincible, Indestructible)

Abhai Abai (Fearless, Unchanging)

Abhoo Ajoo (Unformed, Unborn)

Anaas Akaas (Imperishable, Etheric)

Aganj Abhanj (Unbreakable, Impenetrable)

Alakh Abhakh (Unseen, Unaffected)

Akaal Dyaal (Undying, Merciful)

Alaykh Abhaykh (Indescribable, Uncostumed)

Anaam Akaam (Nameless, Desireless)

Agaahaa Adhaahaa (Unfathomable, Incorruptible)

Anaathay Pramaathay (Unmastered, Destroyer)

Ajonee Amonee (Beyond birth, Beyond silence)

Na Raagay Na Rangay (Beyond love, Beyond colour)

Na Roopay Na Raykay (Beyond form, Beyond shape)

Akaramang Abharamang (Beyond karma, Beyond doubt)

Aganjay Alaykhay (Unconquerable, Indescribable)

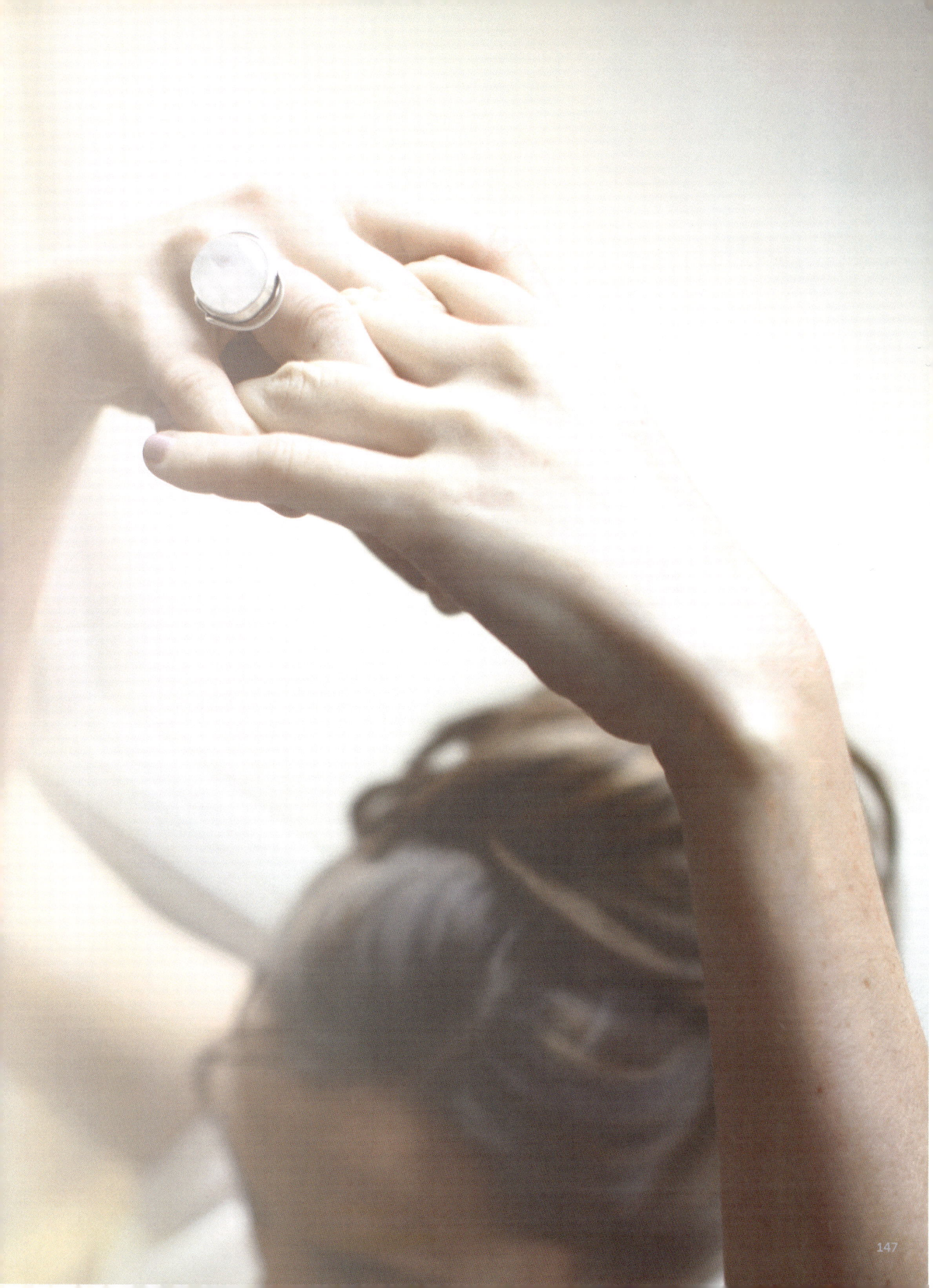

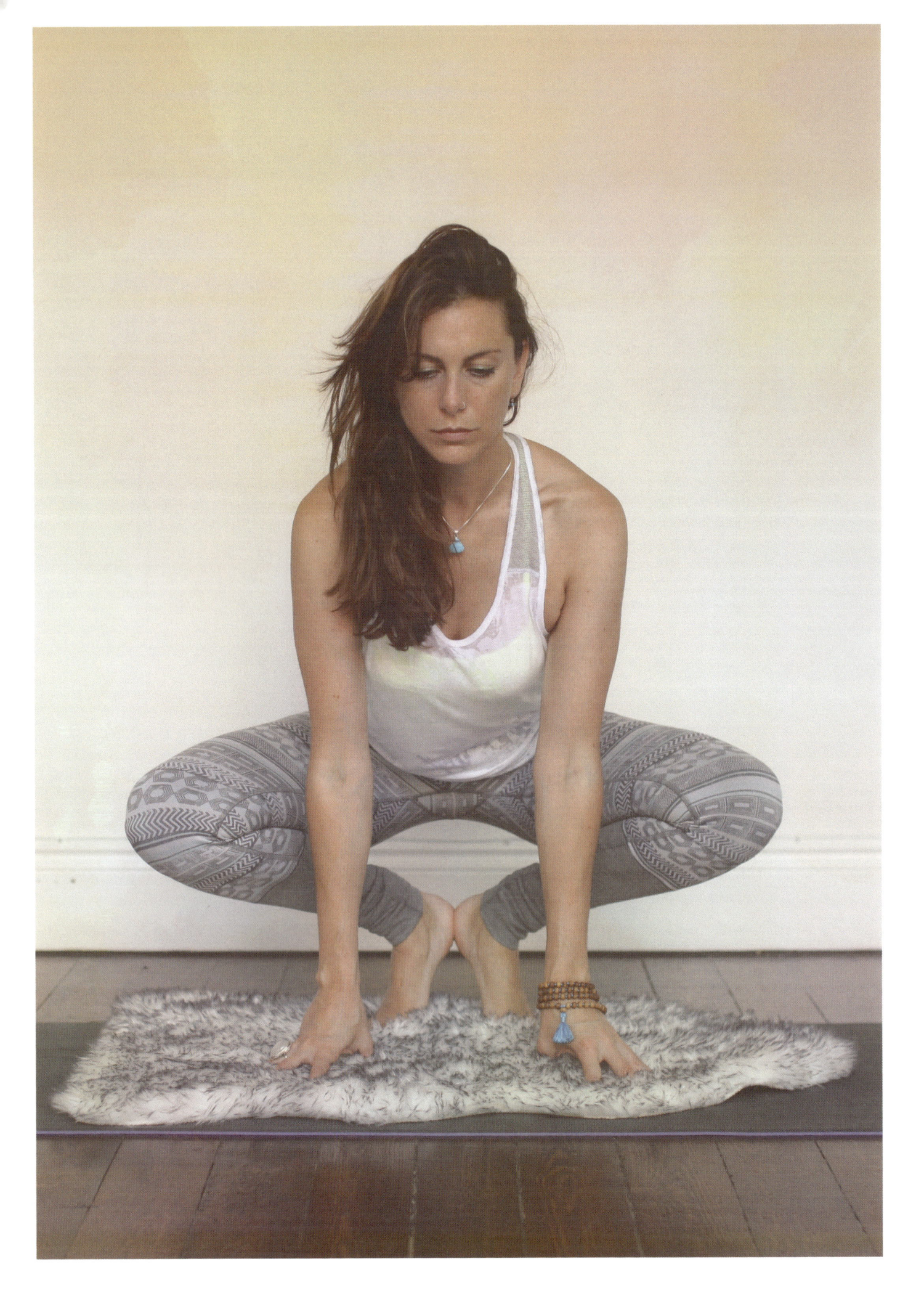

11

ALL-IN-ONE

THE 'I AND I' RELATIONSHIP

Self-realisation through management of The Ten Bodies is incomplete without this additional relationship with The Divine. Without this relationship, you may seek reunion through another individual and return to the Number 2.

#embodyyoursoulpurpose

@roisinallanakiernan

ALL-IN-ONE
THE 'I AND I' RELATIONSHIP

The Number 11 represents two separate and yet inseparable units – the individual and the universal. The little I and the big I. Or 'The I and I', as Rastafaris say. The 'I, with God's help', or 'I, with God-in me'. The 2i in mathematical terms (i+i).

Self-realisation through management of The Ten Bodies is incomplete without this additional relationship with The Divine. It is a relationship or Saint-like way of being that is one with God.

When an individual, complete unit (1) is without relationship with the universal unit (11), it will instead seek reunion through another individual unit (2) – an unfortunate cycle of return.

Despite all the good work that can be done to balance and manage each of your Ten Bodies, there still exists a necessary balance that must be found between individual and divine will. This is the balance that sees you choose situations, people and places you feel are valid for your growth, whilst simultaneously letting go and working with each moment, person and place, as they naturally arise, as they should. It is the interplay of this relationship, between the small I (the individual) and the big I (The Divine), which we can separate in our thinking whilst simultaneously never being separated.

This is a relationship with life that has no difficulty, for it is totally at one and flowing with all that arises.

When you merge your will with The Divine, when you as an individual unit work in parallel union with the universal unit you will find your highest expression, your most-pure, Saint-like way of being - your truest relationship with life.

151

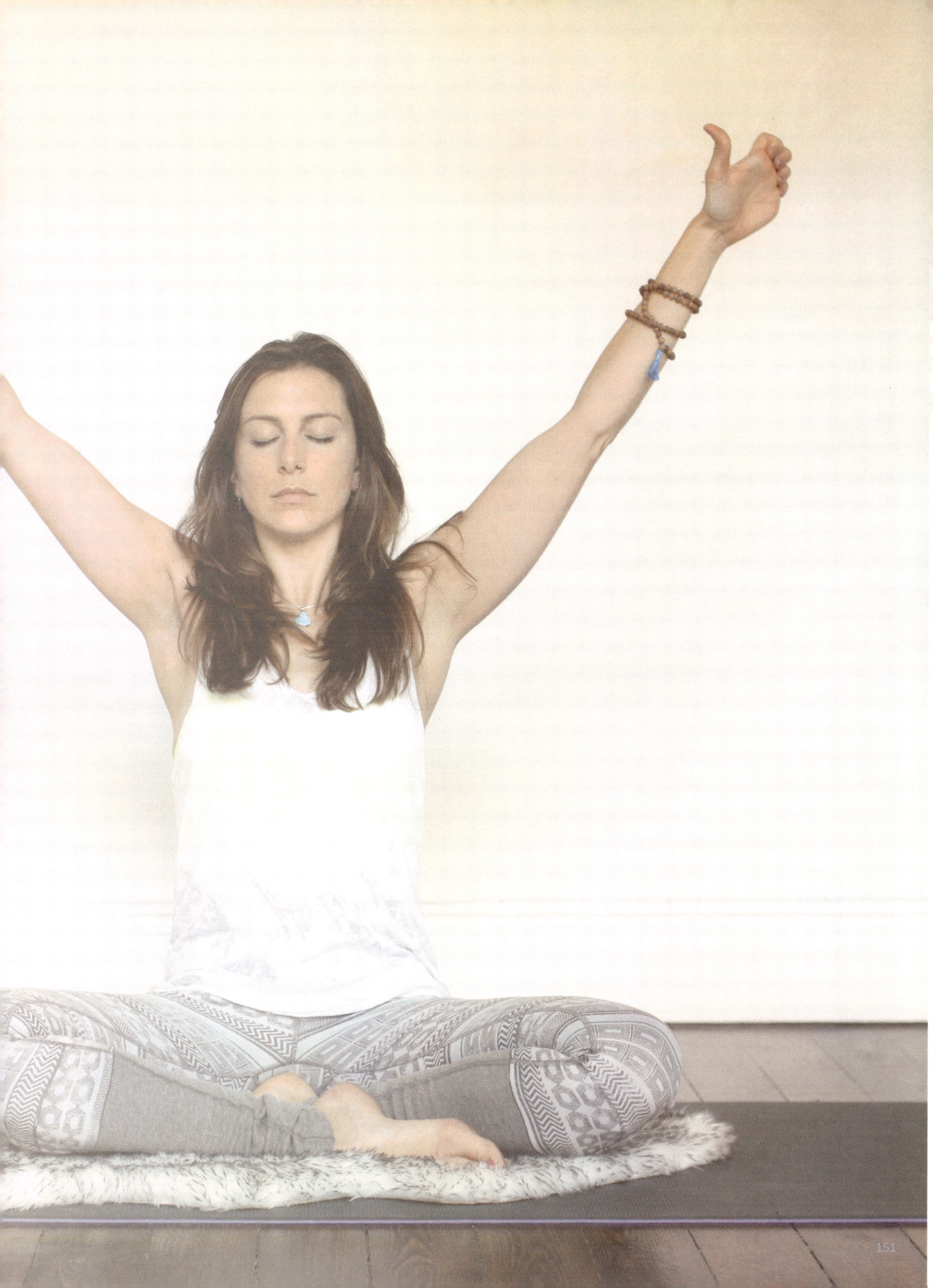

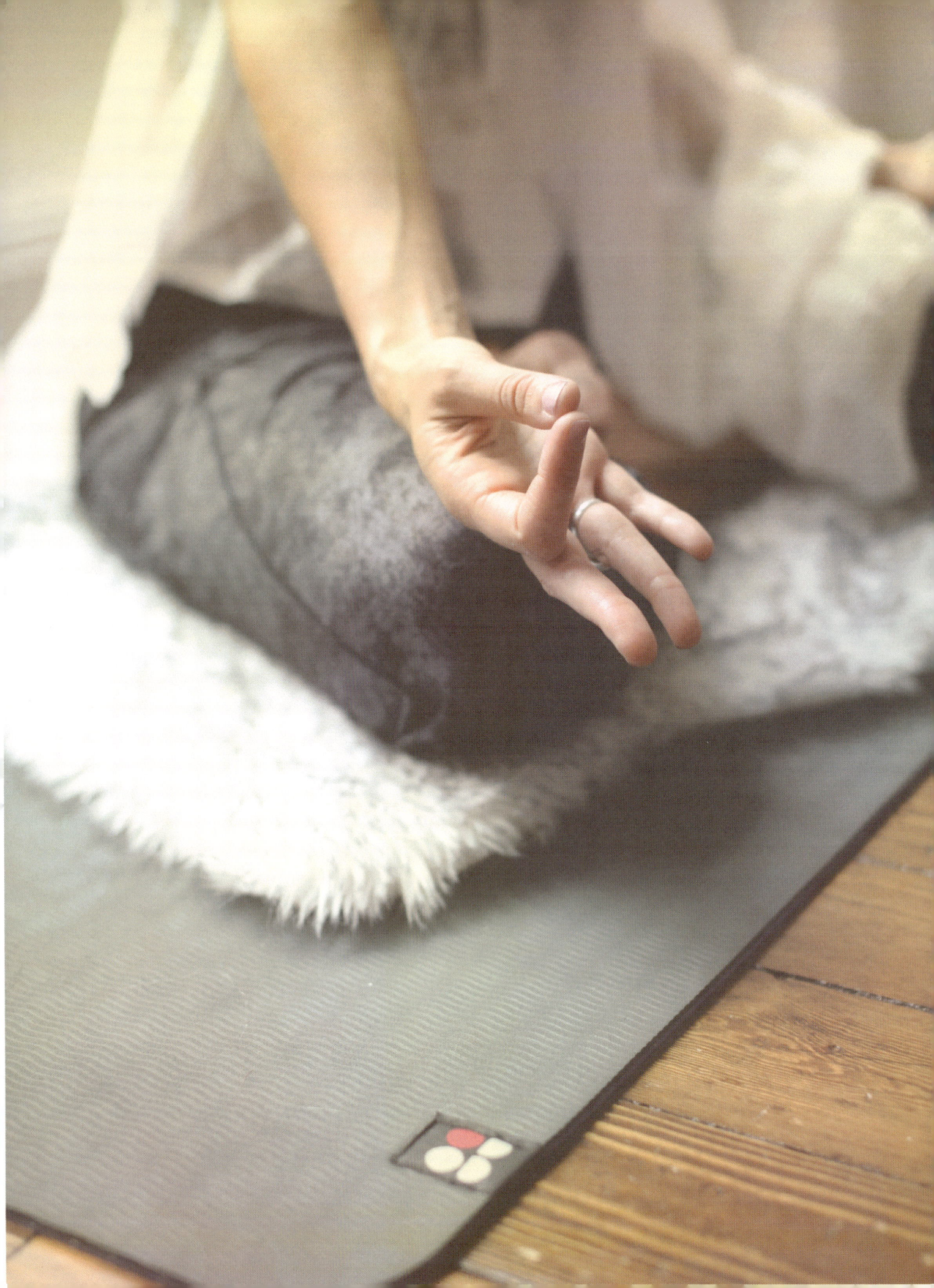

PRANAYAMA

SEVEN-WAVE SAT NAM

POSITION

Sitting with a straight spine, bring your hands into Gyan Mudra (index fingers touching thumbs) on your knees, draw the chin in slightly for a light Jalandhar Bandha, close the eyes and focus in and up between the brows to your Third Eye.

Then, with full awareness, inhale deeply. On the exhale, you're going to vibrate seven 'waves' up through the Chakras. One at the base, two at the sex organs, three at the navel, four at the heart, five at the throat, six at the forehead, and seven out through the top of your head.

As you do this exhaling 'wave', mentally chant 'Sat' (truth) up through your seven chakras, gently pulling the physical area associated with each. Inhale as you mentally chant 'Nam' (name or identity). And continue.

MANTRA

Sat Nam

DURATION

11 - 31 Minutes

COMMENTS

Any sense of separation comes from the mind because we are all divinely connected.

This pranayama meditation activates the part of the brain that's associated with habitual patterns — the mental pathways that keep us locked in thoughts of separation. The bij or seed mantra, Sat Nam (True Name), when used with this seven-wave wash like the sea, cleanses those negative thought processes and brings us in line with our True Identity — our Sat Nam; our Infinite connection.

#embodyyoursoulpurpose
@roisinallanakiernan

KRIYA

AWAKENING TO YOUR TEN BODIES

This kriya brings awareness to each of the Ten Bodies, giving them all a quick tune up and assisting in balance throughout.

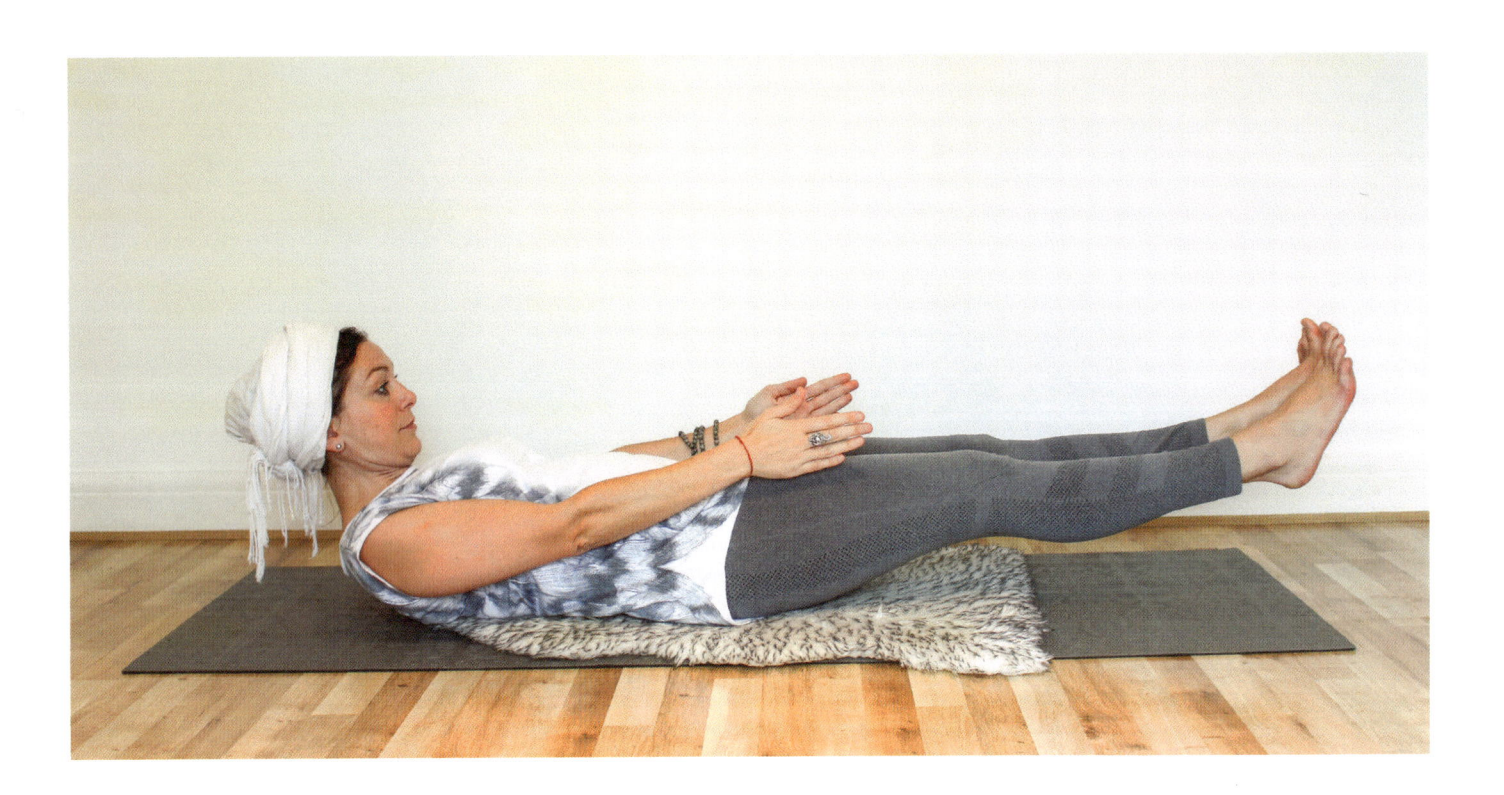

1. Stretch Pose 1-3 Minutes

Instructions: Lying on your back with your arms by your sides, lift the feet together about six inches off the ground – the legs remain straight. Then, reach with your hands (palms facing each other) as if to grab for your feet. Engage your navel and lift the head to also look at your feet – the upper body remains on the mat. Holding this position, use Breath of Fire.

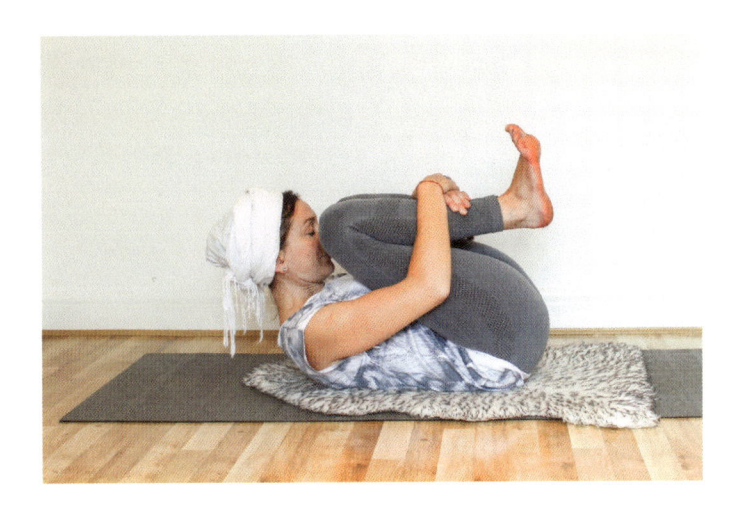

2. Nose to Knees 1-3 Minutes

Instructions: Lying on your back, hug your knees into your chest. Then, engaging the navel again, lift your nose up between your knees and begin Breath of Fire (rapid breathing in and out through the nose using your navel as a pump).

Benefits: These first two exercises will reset the entire nervous system and strengthen the abdominals. The breath is also rejuvenating and purifies the blood.

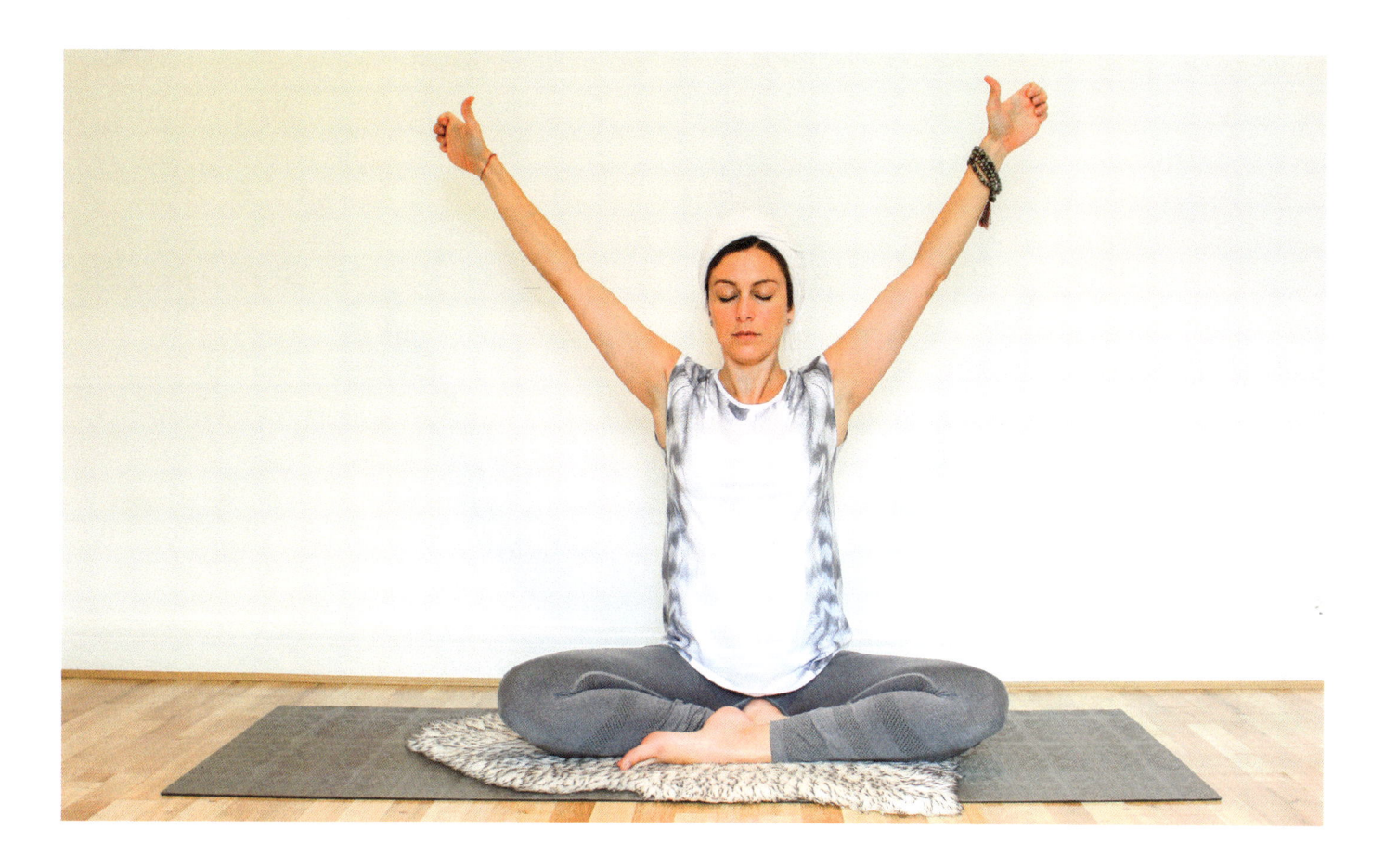

3. Ego Eradicator   1-3 Minutes

Instructions: Sitting tall, place your finger tips on the pads of your hands with the thumbs pulled out to the sides. Then bring your arms up sixty degrees above your head. Close your eyes, concentrate on the space above your head and do Breath of Fire.

To End: Inhale and bring your thumb tips together above your head, hold the position whilst you exhale and apply Mula Bandha (squeezing anal, sexual and navel muscles) then inhale again and relax.

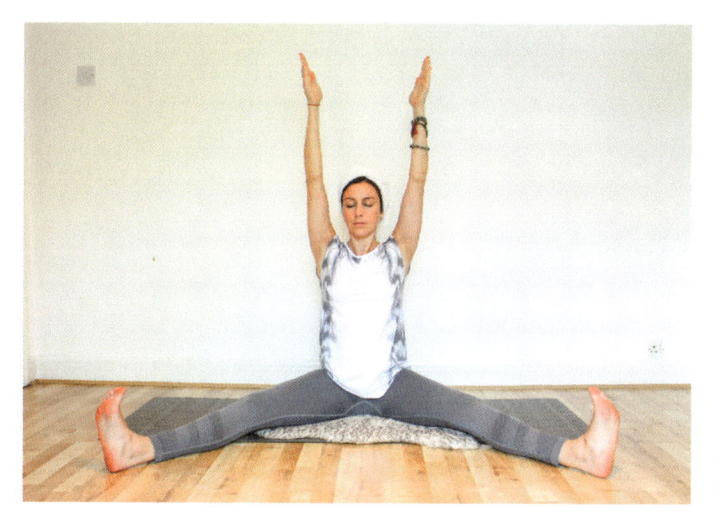

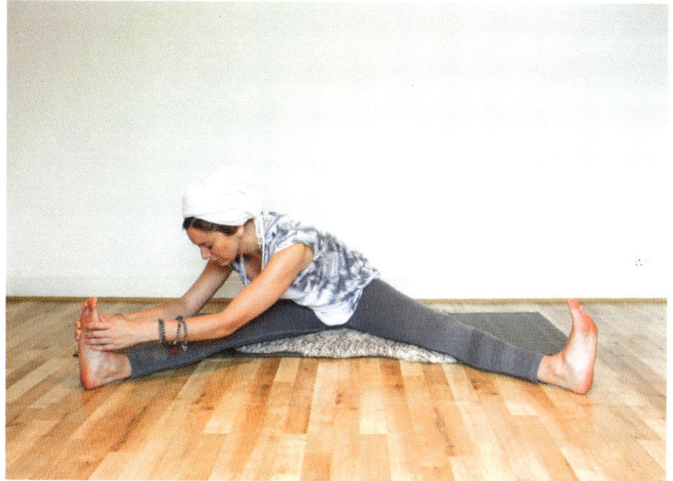

4. Alternating Life Nerve Stretch   2-3 Minutes

Instructions: With your legs stretched out wide in front, inhale your arms straight up above you and then exhale as you fold over each leg in turn – inhale up into the centre and exhale over the legs.

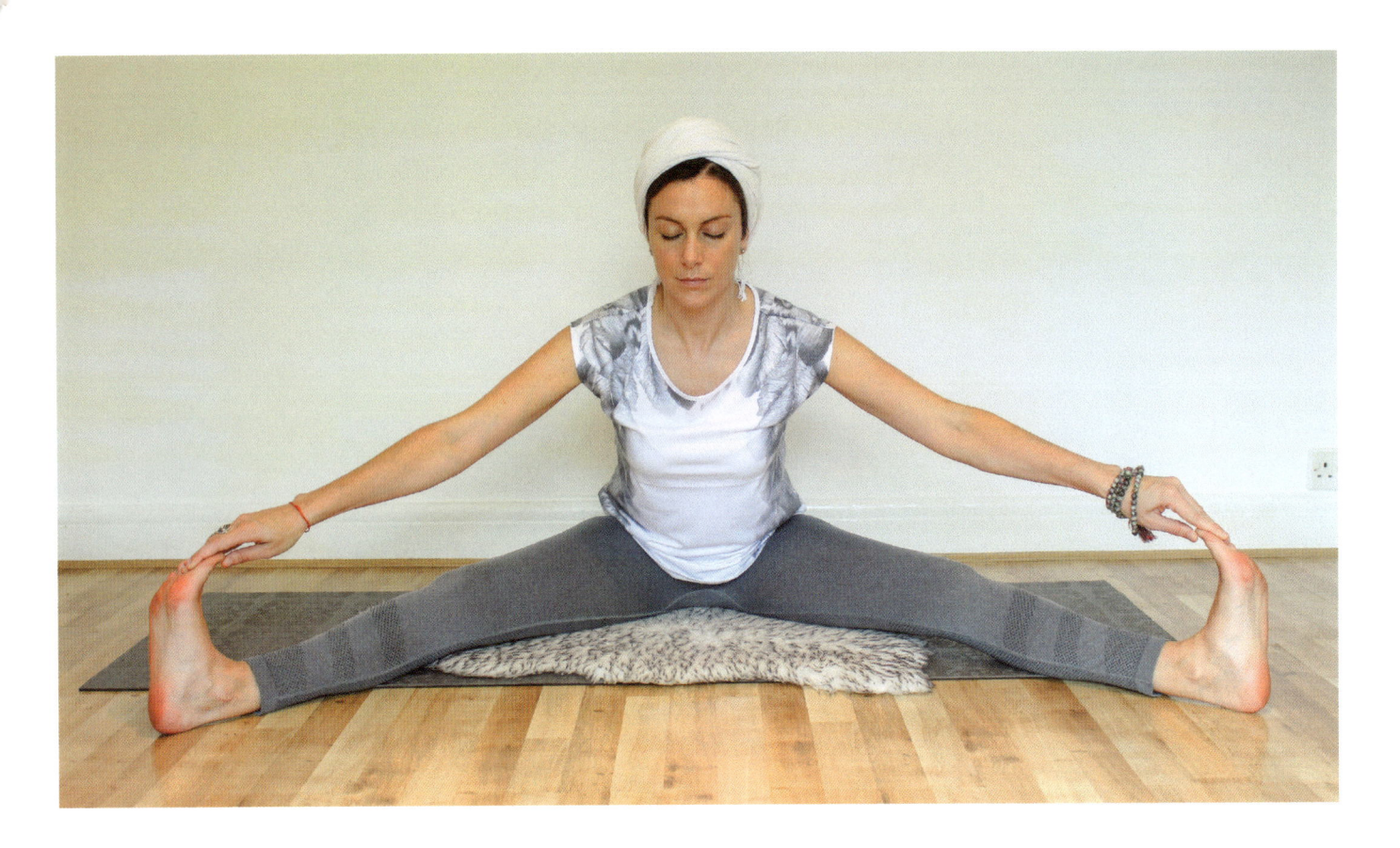

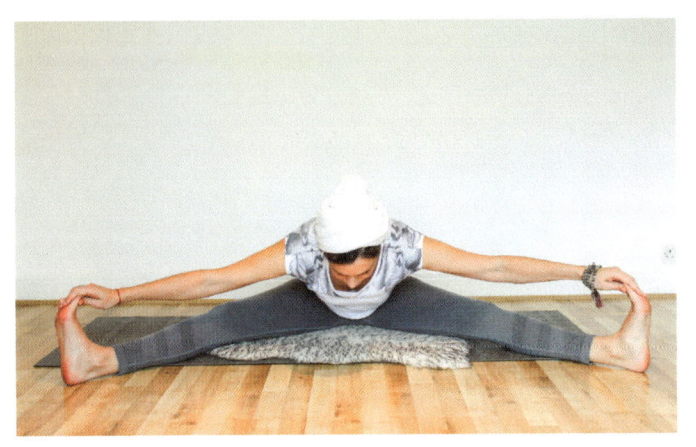

5. Central Life Nerve Stretch 2-3 Minutes

Instructions: Still sitting with your legs wide, reach forward and take hold of the toes of each foot, if you can, otherwise take hold of the leg where you can. Keeping your hold on the toes or leg, inhale as you straighten your spine up and exhale as you fold forward. Continue in this way – inhaling up, exhaling down.

Benefits: Exercises 4&5 predominantly stimulate the sciatic nerves, which are responsible for supplying motor and sensory information to the legs.

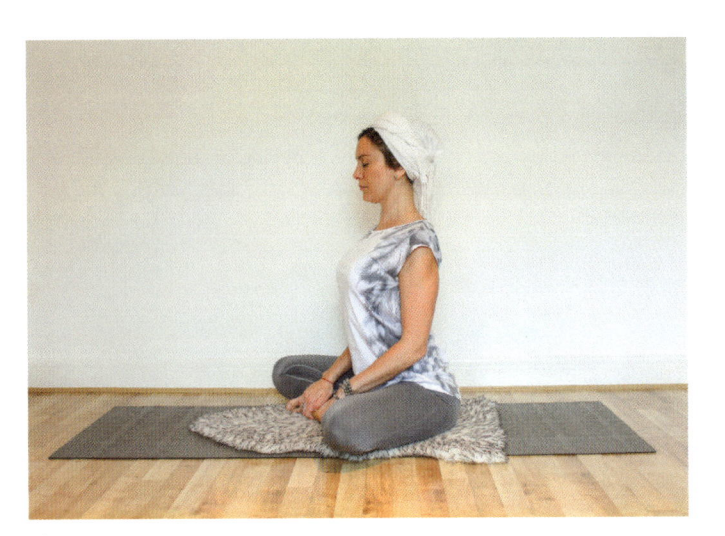

6. Spinal Flex 1-3 Minutes

Instructions: Sitting tall with the legs crossed take hold of your shins and, keeping the head in line with the base of your spine, inhale as you arch your torso forward (opening chest and shoulders) and exhale as you round back. The head doesn't move.

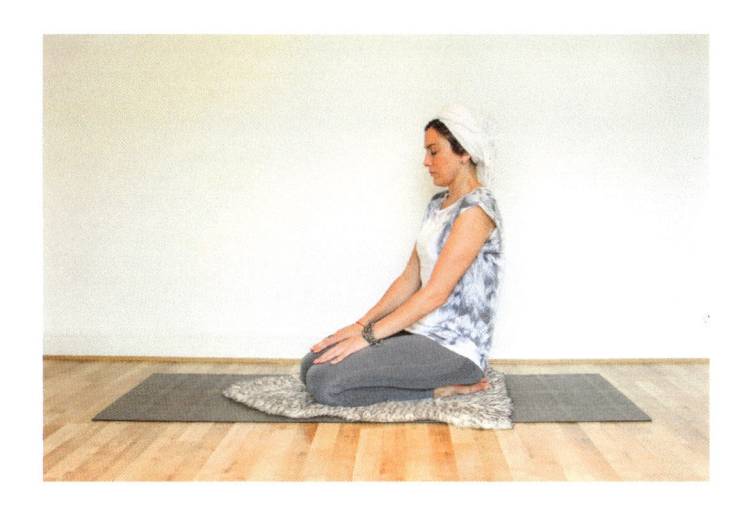

7. Spinal Flex on the Knees 1-3 Minutes

Instructions: Sitting on the heels, place your hands flat on the thighs and continue the Spinal Flex exercise as before – inhaling the torso forward, exhaling it back and keeping the head in line with the base of the spine. Focus on the Third Eye (in and up between the brows).

Benefits: This works to bring strength and flexibility to the lower back. After 3 minutes, the brain wave patterns change, making you more calm.

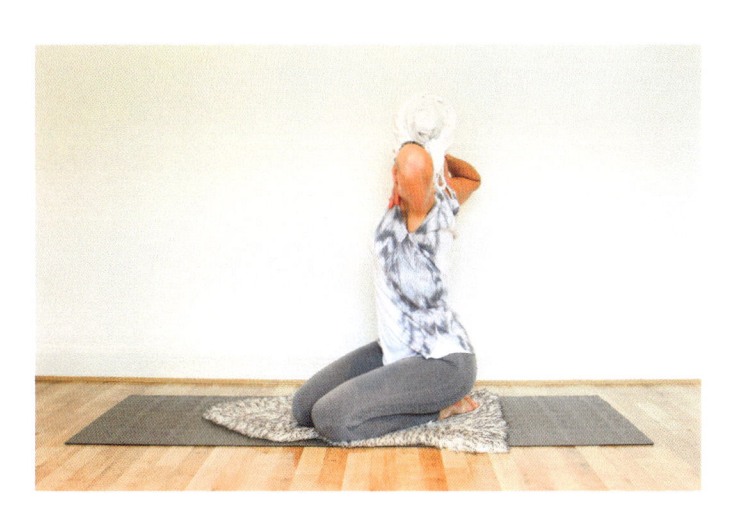

8. Spinal Twist on the Knees 1-3 Minutes

Instructions: Stay on your knees but take hold of the shoulders this time – fingers in front, thumbs behind. Let the head follow the flow of the body now. Inhaling as you twist left, exhaling as you twist right. Keep your elbows up in line with your shoulders.

Benefits: This works to stretch and tone the upper back, whilst the twist is detoxifying.

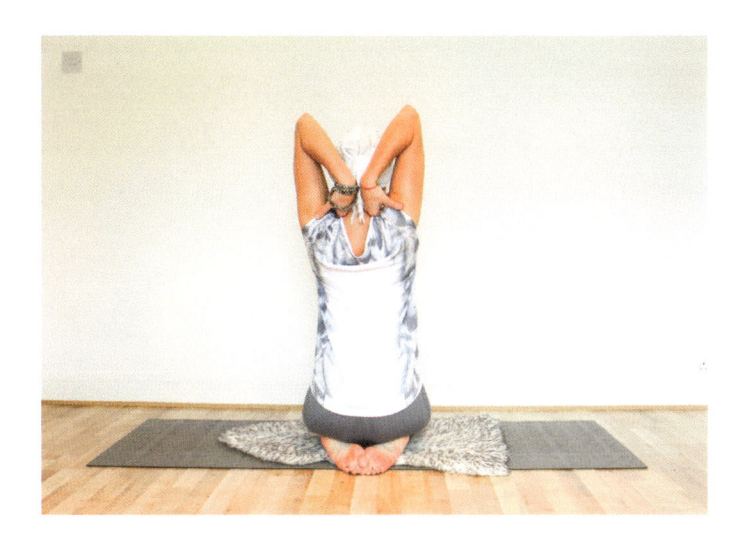

9. Elbow Lifts 1-3 Minutes

Instructions: Still holding on to the shoulders as in the last exercise, now you're going to inhale and bring the backs of the hands together behind your head and then exhale down.

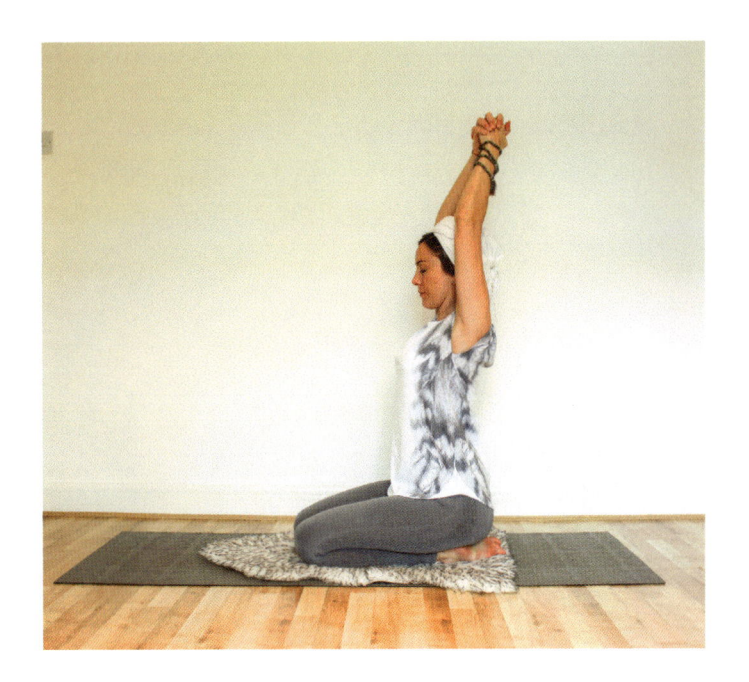

10. Arm Pumps 1-3 Minutes

Instructions: Still sitting on the heels, interlace your fingers in Venus Lock in front of you and inhale as you stretch them up in front, exhale down. Keep your arms straight throughout.

Benefits: As well as toning the arms, I like to think of this exercise as a tangible exercise to cut through the crap you carry.

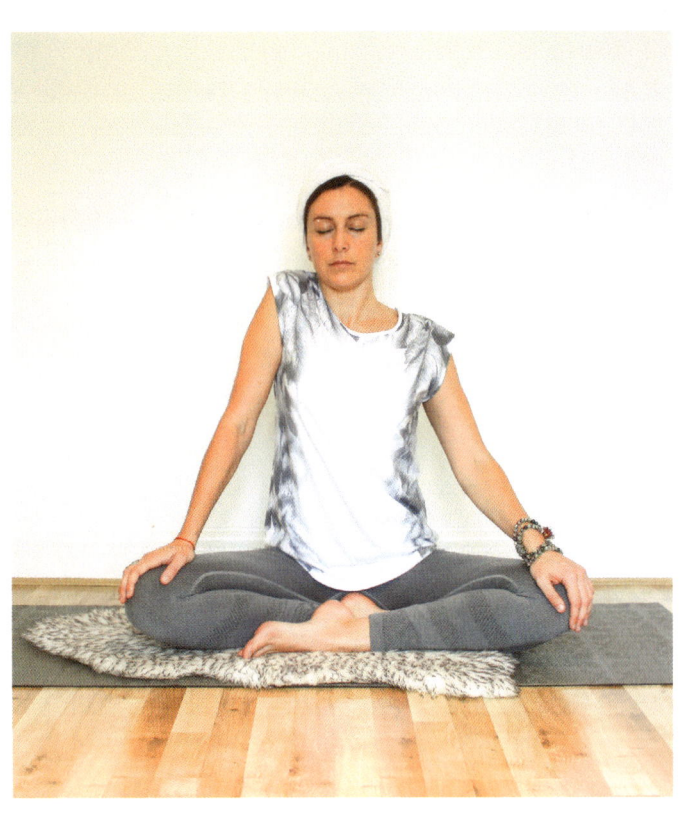

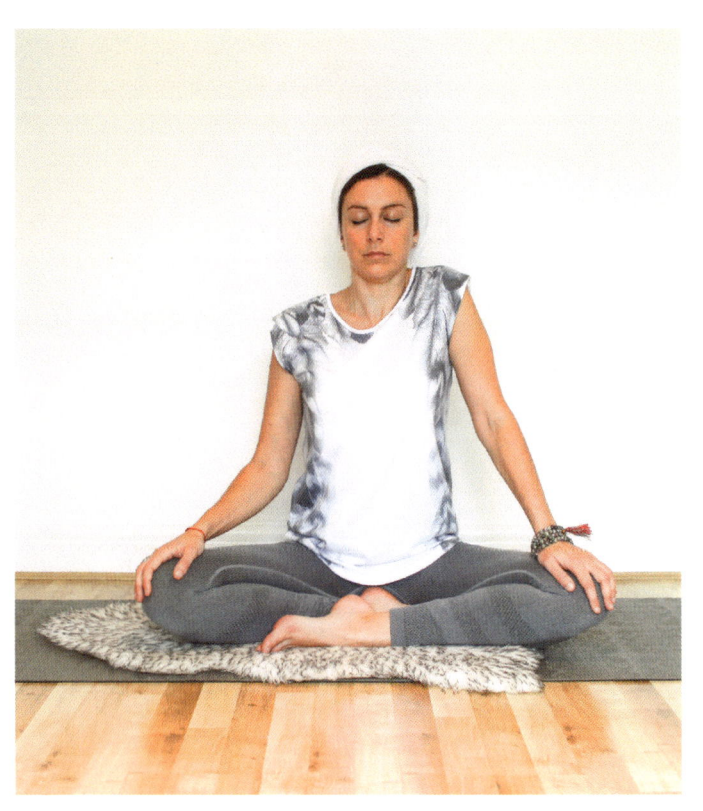

11. Alternating Shoulder Shrugs 1 Minute Each Side

Instructions: Sitting with your spine tall, rest your hands on your knees and inhale the left shoulder up then, as you exhale, your right shoulder comes up and your left goes down.

Continue for one minute then move in the opposite direction for a minute – inhaling right to start.

12. Double Shoulder Shrugs 1 Minutes

Instructions: Sitting as before, simply inhale both shoulders up and then exhale both shoulders down.

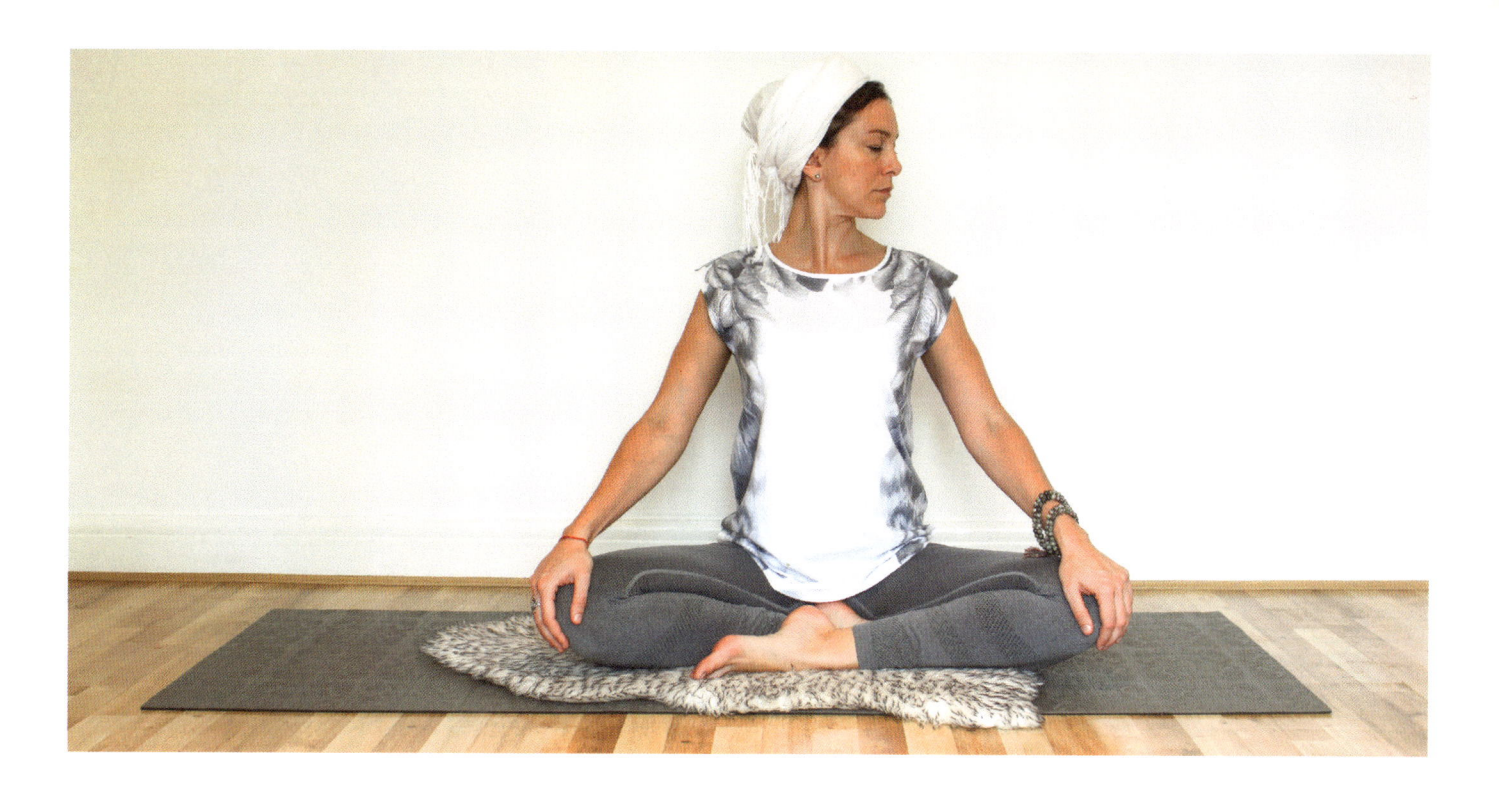

13. Neck Turns 1 Minute Each Side

Instructions: Sitting with a tall spine, inhale as you turn your head to the left then exhale as you turn right. Speed up so it becomes like a 'no' head shake.

Then reverse the breath and head shake.

To End: Inhale, suspend the breath, focus at the Third Eye and then slowly exhale.

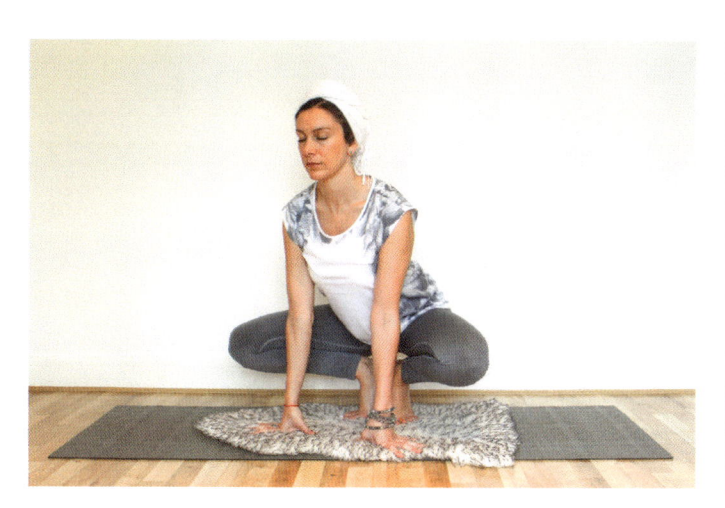

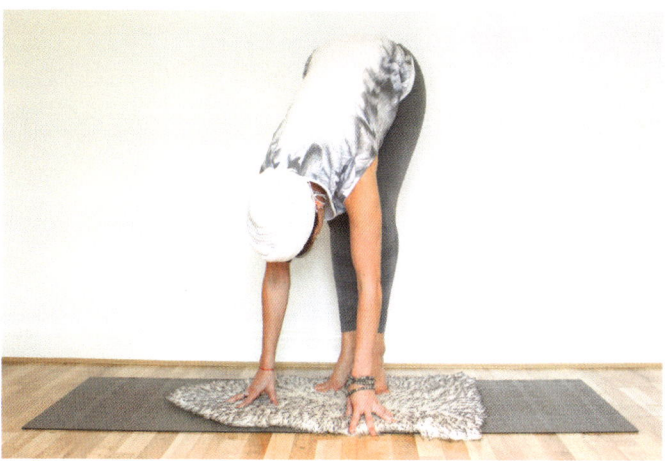

14. Frog Pose 26 - 54 Reps

Instructions: From standing, squat down so your buttocks are on the heels. Ideally, both heels will be off the ground and together with the toes turned out, your hands rest on the floor in front and your face looks forward – frog pose. From there you're going to inhale as you straighten the legs – the heels remain off the ground and your head drops down. Continue then, inhaling up, exhaling down.

MEDITATION
LAYA YOGA

POSITION

Sit with a tall spine and the hands active on the knees in Gyan Mudra (back of the wrists on the knees, palms facing forward with the index fingers touching thumbs).

We're going to chant a three and a half cycle mantra, which is the same rhythm as the flow of the Kundalini energy. So, as you chant, imagine it spiralling up from the base of your spine to the top of your head.

MANTRA

Ek Ong Kar (uh)
Sa Ta Na Ma (uh)
Siree Wha (uh)
Hay Guru

MEANING

The Creator and the Creation are One. This is our True Identity. The ecstasy of the experience of this wisdom is beyond all words and brings indescribable bliss.

FURTHER DIRECTIONS

On 'Ek' pull the navel in and on each 'uh' lift the diaphragm up firmly. The 'uh' is more of a powerful movement than a sound. When it comes to 'Hay Guru' relax the navel and abdomen.

The eyes are nine tenths closed and your attention is at the Third Eye.

DURATION

11 - 31 Minutes

TO END

Inhale deeply and hold the breath as long as you can before exhaling and relaxing.

#embodyyoursoulpurpose
@roisinallanakiernan

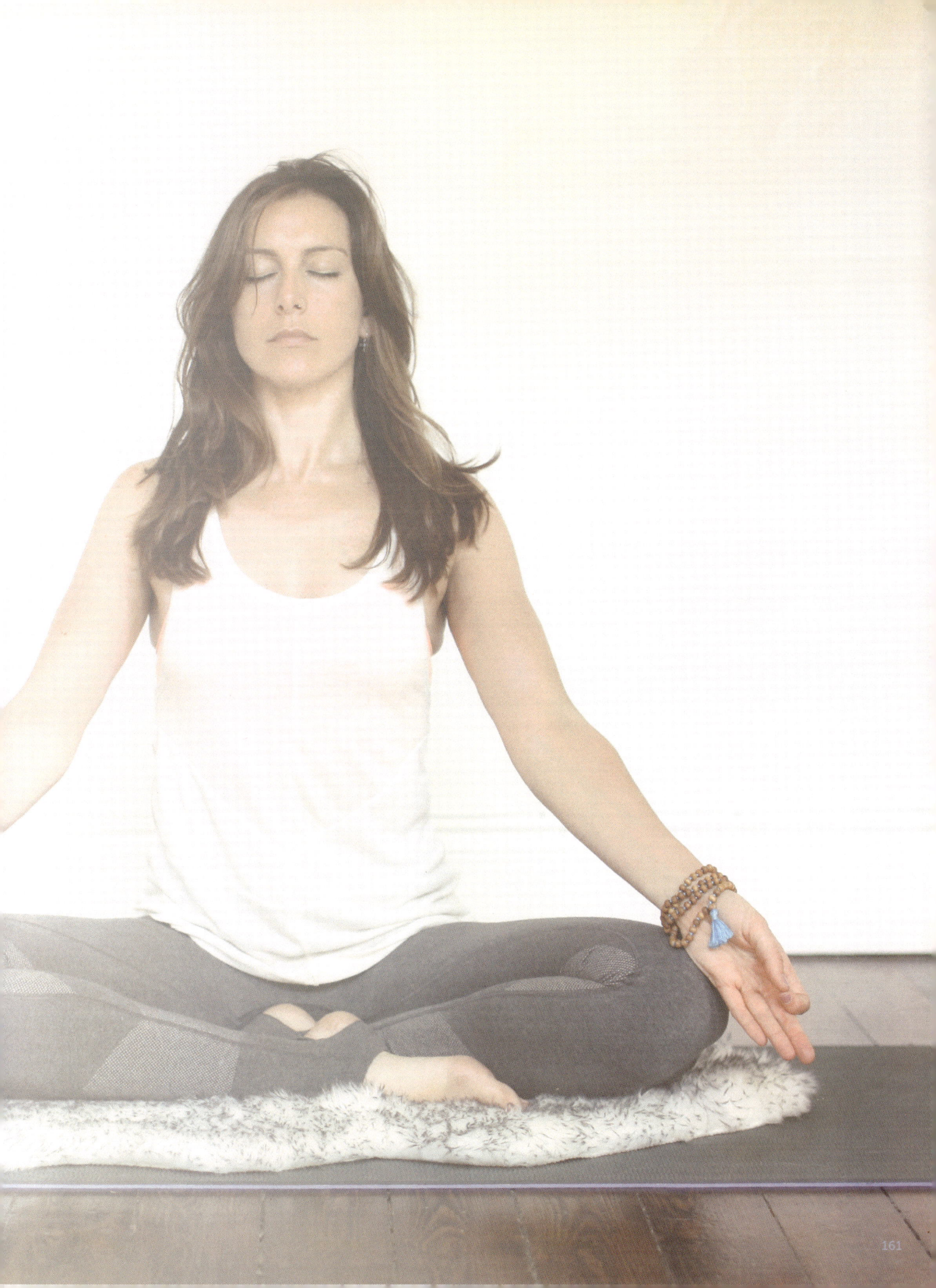

ABOUT THE AUTHOR

I like to call myself a Mystic Gypsy!

Born and bred in London, I have Celtic roots, and a free-spirited nature. As a child I wanted to be a nun, until I read into Catholicism and found boys, clothes and parties. I could also hear a louder voice of encouragement, calling me to follow society's steps to so-called success. Like all of life, though, it went full circle.

I'd spent years working day and night to build a career as a journalist. I did well too – my work has been published in The Independent, The Mirror, Conde Nast Traveller, Cosmopolitan Magazine, FHM, Yoga Magazine and Om Yoga Magazine. Then, in 2008, my Mum died. Dad was in hospital at the same time and died a few years later. Both were sensitive, damaged souls that were drawn together then pulled apart by their pain. I'd tried their method of escape during my teens and knew it didn't work, so I tried feeling and used my parents' lives as lessons for growth. Their deaths made me realise how short life can be and that mine needed to change. So, I trained as a Kundalini Yoga teacher and started to write my first novel. I'd been practicing yoga since my teen's and writing creatively for as long as I could remember. My career as a journalist no longer fit. I wanted to live life for me – to share what I enjoyed doing, not just follow a money-making path in something similar.

My focus now is more to do with Tantra, especially the Sexual Shamanic practises offered via the International School of Temple Arts (ISTA). I also work closely with women in this field, supporting them to reclaim their inner power via Kundalini Yoga, Tantra, and Sexual Shamanism. As part of this, I've recently been taken on as Global Organiser for the Women Who See In The Dark movement, which supports women to own their victim/shadow stories, as well as their inner masculine.

My aim is to encourage others to listen to the stirrings of their own souls and start to live their truth – start to embody their soul purpose. I truly believe that it's imperative, in this paradoxical age of disconnection despite global connection, that people start tuning in to their feelings – rather than numbing and escaping. Regardless of societal, familial or peer-driven expectations, I encourage people to reconnect within, really listen (to themselves and others), find a way to release negative patterns and do more of what makes them truly happy.

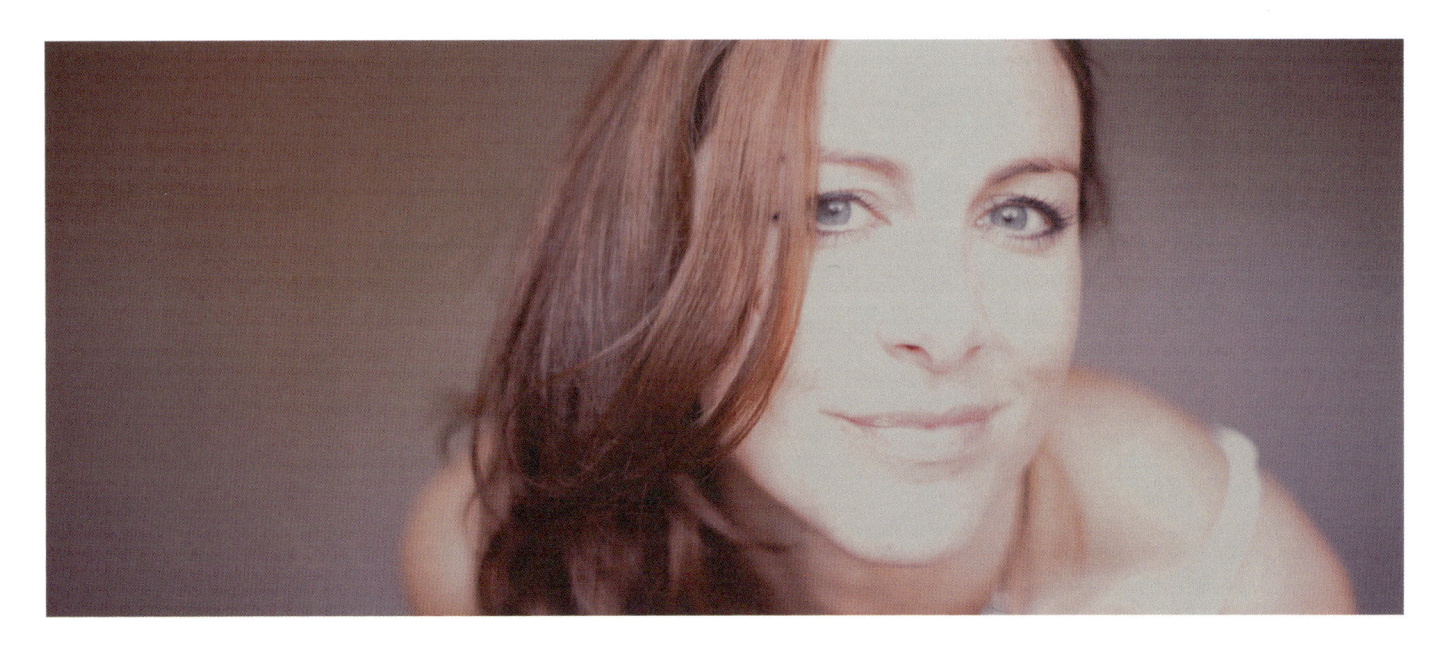

QUICK REFERENCE GUIDE

1. The Soul Body
HEAD OR HEART

Your infinite, all-connected essence – the true you, whispered through your heart's desires. When out of balance, you'll come more from your head than your heart.

2. The Protective (Negative) Mind
DIVISION OR UNITY

When out of balance, you'll be over-protective or negative, clinging on to people or situations as a method of control. Relationships (shown through the number 2) are important to this body.

3. The Projective (Positive) Mind
BALANCE INDIVIDUAL WILL WITH DIVINE WILL

A positive mental attitude helps us to achieve but then we must learn to trust and let go, with good humour, secure in the knowledge that all will work out as it should.

4. The Meditative (Neutral) Mind
BREATHE, THEN ACT

A meditative mind will 'tick-tock' between the pros and cons of each situation and find a place of neutrality between them.

5. The Physical Body
COMMUNICATION INCLUDES LISTENING

Five is the half way point to ten – the bridge, or communicative link; the teacher. Are you participating fully – receiving all messages and responding in service, for others and yourself?

6. The Arcline
WORRIER OR WARRIOR

Your halo, symbolised by a sword, which can be pointed at you (worry) or away from you (warrior). What you put out, or point towards yourself, all depends on you. Strengthen the subtleties of this body to alert and guide you with integrity.

7. The Aura
BAGGAGE OR ELEVATION

The magnetic field that surrounds your body can either trap you in patterns of reaction (your baggage) or bring awareness to protect and uplift in each moment with transparency.

8. The Pranic Body
THE INFINITE BREATH

Prana is the life force energy we take in through the breath, which flows in and out like the tide, coming and going, moment to moment. We can either flow with it or create resistance through fear and control, leading to illness.

9. The Subtle Body
MYSTERY OR MASTERY

Go deep into the core of you by staying put and focussing with discernment, discipline and patience. In this way you can choose mastery over your life, rather than circling the mystery.

10. The Radiant Body
ALL OR NOTHING

The combination of this 1 (Soul Body) with 0 can either offer infinite completion for the soul's journey or a removal of connection. You can either feel courageous or fearful; aspirational or unmotivated; confident or lacking self-esteem.

11. All-in-one
THE 'I AND I' RELATIONSHIP

Self-realisation through management of The Ten Bodies is incomplete without this additional relationship with The Divine. Without this relationship, you may seek reunion through another individual and return to the Number 2.

RESOURCES

Much of the wisdom shared in this book comes from Yogi Bhajan's teachings of Kundalini Yoga – the dates and sources of which are listed here.

Also of note is the expanded 'Tree of Life' knowledge, which descends from Shiv Charan Singh, in association with Yogi Bhajan's teaching on The Ten Bodies. Shiv calls his life's work Karam Kriya - 'Total action through which our karma is brought to completion through application of spiritual consciousness guided by the intelligence of numbers,' (www.karamkriya.com).

BOOKS FROM SHIV CHARAN SINGH:

- Let The Numbers Guide You. The Spiritual Science of Numerology.
- Tantric Numerology, Science of Soul Mastery.
- Try Thinking of it This Way.

The Yogi Bhajan image on p.10 is from 1985 and shared via Creative Commons Attribution-Share Alike 4.0 International. The original copyright is owned by the Kundalini Research Institute. (https://en.wikipedia.org/wiki/Harbhajan_Singh_Khalsa#/media/File:Yogi_Bhajan_1985.jpg)

Regarding the date December 21, 2012, noted on page.10 'About Kundalini Yoga', I suggest exploring online. A good place to start would be Wikipedia, which offers several references and ongoing exploration - https://en.wikipedia.org/wiki/2012_phenomenon

PRANAYAMAS AND MEDITATIONS:

- For a calm heart (TT L1 Manual p.69, September 1981)
- Balancing mind and heart unto infinity (Transformation vol. 2, p.6 April 4, 1972)
- For the negative mind (The Mind: Its Projections and Multiple Facets, p.153)
- For the positive mind (The Mind: Its Projections and Multiple Facets, p.154)
- Shabd Kriya (Kundalini Manual for Intermediate students, p.50, April 1, 1974)
- Dhrib Dhrishti Lochina Karma (3HO website - Reprinted from Aquarian Times, Summer 2003 https://www.3ho.org/kundalini-yoga/meditation/featured-meditations/dhrib-dhrishti-lochina-karma-meditation-inspiring)
- For the Arcline and to clear the karmas (The Master's Touch, p.208, August 1, 1996)
- Divine Shield Meditation (TT L1 Manual, p.92, September 1971)
- Hunsani Meditation on the white swan (Kundalini Manual for Intermediate students, p.41, January 13, 1975)
- To clarify the subtle body (Praana Praanee Praanayam, p.150, October 11, 1996)
- Antar Naad Mudra (TT L1 Manual p.86)
- To develop the radiant body (I Am A Woman p.38, July 31, 2001)
- Seven wave Sat Nam (TT L1 Manual p.123)

KRIYAS:

- KY for balancing head and heart (KY for Youth and Joy, Shakta Kaur Khalsa, p 92-93)
- Meditation to Open the Lock of the Heart and Increase the Power of the Infinite Within (I Am A Woman, Sat Purkh Kaur Khalsa, editor, p. 92)
- For the negative mind (The Ten Light Bodies of Consciousness, Nirvair Singh, p.45-51)
- For the positive mind (Waves of Healing by Siri Atma Singh, p.136 -145)
- For the fourth body (The Ten Light Bodies of Consciousness, Nirvair Singh, p.84-86)
- Foundation for Infinity (TT L1 Manual , p.31-32)
- Adjust your flow with The Four U's (I Am A Woman p.194, July 5, 1984)
- For S.A.D and Depression (The Art, Science and Application of KY)
- Preparatory exercises for lungs, magnetic field and deep meditation (TT L1 Manual p.40-41, November 27, 1974)
- Laya Yoga Kriya – for intuition and the power to heal (TT L1 Manual, p.101)
- For the radiant Body (Waves of Healing by Siri Atma Singh, p.222 -227)
- Awakening To Your Ten Bodies (TT L1 Manual p.11-12)

GLOSSARY

Bandha

One of three interior energy locks, created by squeezing muscles within the body.

These are great for helping you to sustain a pose as it supports you from the inside. They also help to regulate and control all your internal systems – hormonal, sexual, metabolic, digestive and so on.

Mula Bandha

Also known as root lock, this energy lock is formed by squeezing anal, sexual and navel muscles together. It's used a lot in Kundalini Yoga as it stimulates the pelvic nerves and genital system, where your sacred, sexual energy – the Kundalini - is based. This lock also stimulates the excretory system so is good for relieving constipation and depression.

Uddiyana Bandha

Also known as flying up lock, it's done by drawing your diaphragm, stomach and abdominals up into the rib cage, thereby lifting your energy up. This lock offers great relief for any abdominal or stomach problems. The adrenals are also balanced with this lock, offering relief from stress, lethargy and tension. And it's good for increasing your metabolism and toning abdominals.

Note that the breath should be equal in strength and length; both the inhale and exhale. The optimum rhythm is 2-3 cycles per second.

Jalandhar Bandha

This is throat lock, which controls the flow of energy in the nerves and blood vessels of the neck. You simply tuck your chin in until you feel a lengthening along the back of your neck. It works by compressing the sinuses on the main arteries of the neck, which helps to regulate the circulatory and respiratory systems. It also balances the thyroid and metabolism. And is an instant stress and anger reliever.

Mudra

An exterior energy seal, used by connecting the hands or fingers in a specific way. These work to relax the brain and guide the flow of energy.

Gyan Mudra

Index or Jupiter finger touching thumb – a seal of knowledge and ability; of receptivity and calm. The thumb represents the ego.

Buddhi Mudra

Baby or Mercury finger touching thumb – for clear and intuitive communication.

Prayer Mudra

Both hands pressed firmly together, neutralising the masculine and feminine energies, as well as the hemispheres of the brain.

Pranayama

This literally means breath control. Prana is the breath or life force energy and Yama means to control. They're breathing exercises basically.

Venus Lock

Interlace your fingers. Men, left thumb on top. Women, right thumb on top. This channels sexual energy, promotes glandular balance, and develops the ability to concentrate easily. The mounds at the base of the thumbs represent Venus; sensuality and sexuality. The thumb represents the ego.

Third Eye

This is really your sixth chakra – the Ajna; the seat of your intuition. It helps you to see without the eyes. To know.

Breath of Fire

This breathing exercise or pranayama is used a lot in Kundalini Yoga. It's done by breathing rapidly in and out through the nose, using the navel as a pump to draw the breath in and push it back out. It's a rhythm a bit like a dog panting, or you sniffing, as opposed to long deep breathing. A tip to remember is that if you find yourself gasping for more air then you're going too fast. Take it slow at first and build it up – it takes some getting used to.

Pregnant ladies (beyond 4months), those with blood pressure problems and anyone under the age of 16 should refrain from using this powerful breathing exercise.

It works to oxygenate and purify blood; flushes out toxins from the organs; stimulates the energy channels of the body; enhances any pose; brings the glands into balance; and strengthens the magnetic field or Aura.

Long, Deep Breathing

Many people oversee this fundamental breath but its benefits are numerous and can be taken into everyday life. Breathing through each of the three chambers of the lungs – abdominal or lower, chest or middle and clavicular or upper – can enhance your life. Full, deep breathing helps to relax and calm you, due to its influence on the parasympathetic nervous system. It detoxifies the system. Stimulates the brain chemicals – endorphins – that fight depression. Cleanses the blood and therefore organs. Regulates the body's PH system. Increases energy and vitality. And helps you to manage your emotions and therefore actions.

Chakra

The chakras are energy centres within the body – areas that relate to different organs, development stages and emotions. In the tantric Kundalini system of Chakras we look at seven up through the body and an eighth – The Aura.

Mantra

Mantra literally means mind distraction – it helps to focus your mind in meditation, so you can relax. A mantra can simply be an affirmation – something you continuously say to yourself to re-condition your beliefs. In Kundalini Yoga we mostly use mantras from the Sikh holy book, which is in a language called Gurmukhi. This language was created resonantly, rather than contextually like our language, and so it works to 'key' at 84 reflex points in the roof of the mouth and 'pluck' at the 74,000 nadis or energy channels that run from the stomach.

Printed in Great Britain
by Amazon